ACUPUNCTURISTS
MEAN BUSINESS

A guide to creating a prospering and profitable acupuncture practice.

Published by

Katie Altneu, L.Ac. MSOM FABORM

www.acuprosper.com

For Worldwide Distribution, Printed in the U.S.A.

ISBN: 978-0-578-61996-5

Dedicated to a world in need of harmony and balance and the healers devoted to helping them find it.

Table of Contents

Introduction

Congratulations! Whether you're a rookie acupuncturist, an acupuncture student, or a seasoned acupuncturist with many years under your belt – I want to give you a huge high five and a bow of respect.

You are amazing. You have mastered a complex, mysterious, and potent medicine. You can speak biomed and Chinese med; discern the underlying roots of problems and recognize western pathology; map anatomy, muscles, and tendons as well as energetic pathways; address the physical body as well as the spirit; treat your patients with confident authority and compassionately hold space for them.

All of the above is what makes acupuncturists so remarkable and important; we are practicing in a time when modern science, doctors, and physical therapists are trying to catch up with, explain, and even borrow from our ancient medicine. As acupuncturists, our job is to cultivate a mutual understanding and respect between ourselves and modern medicine while holding fast to our ancient roots and principles. Acupuncture is incredible, deep, and diverse in its application. With it, you have a very powerful set of tools that will allow you to transform lives for the better.

I want to thank you for carrying this torch. This is not to be taken lightly. It can be daunting when patients look to you to solve and relieve their complicated health problems. And it's daunting to find yourself in the role of small business owner, or as I like to call it, acupreneur. You have been called to this profession for a reason. A beautiful reason: I believe there are people you're meant to serve. And I believe you can change the world.

The world needs acupuncture now more than ever. Our health care system is struggling. In addition to a rise in chronic ailments, there's an epidemic of pain disorders, addiction, and anxiety. Acupuncture is well-equipped to help all of these things. Our practices should be bustling and yours can be. Yet so many are struggling. Which makes me sad, and is why I am writing this book.

Not only does this profession need competent acupuncturists, it needs competent and *confident* acupuncturists who know how to heal their patients while effectively communicating about our medicine and the value it provides. It needs acupuncturists who know how to get their message heard by the people who need to hear it. It needs acupuncturists who are willing to stand up, lead, be courageous, and be heard.

We need to show the world that we mean business.

We need to show the world that we, and our medicine, demand respect. But here's the thing: One can't simply *demand* respect. It's something that must be *inspired*.

To understand how to effectively inspire respect, you must first understand that there's a wrong way to go about it. We don't decry other health practitioners. We don't devalue our services, time, education, and ability to provide transformative results by offering rates that are too low. We don't operate in dinky, dusty clinics or with outdated websites. And we don't guarantee that acupuncture is an energy medicine that "fixes everything."

We inspire respect by meeting potential clients and professional peers at their personal levels and explaining how our medicine can help them in a way they'll understand. By valuing and honoring our services. By having professional offices and websites. By being an absolute pleasure to do business with. By knowing how to communicate about our medicine.

While what our profession could really use is a million-dollar PR campaign like *Got Milk?* Or *Beef. It's What's for Dinner.* Without the lofty budget required for such a campaign (please go join your state association if you're not already a member, by the way), we're each left to do it for ourselves. Our job is to find creative ways to market our practices and educate our community about how we can help. Acupuncturists must master the art of communicating about our medicine and be prepared to run "grassroots" PR and public health education campaigns that get our audience shaking their heads in a resounding "yes". That's good marketing and good business, and you can learn it. I'm hoping this book will help you to do this.

My Story, briefly

I'm an acupuncturist and herbalist with a clinic in Denver. I opened my clinic in 2011, and within less than five years, grew to have a waitlist, several associates on staff and an online fertility course. I want to tell you that I don't see five million people a day; spending time with my patients is really important to me. And I don't work a million hours a week - my work-life-balance is also really important to me. I'm a new mom. And I don't have multiple locations, because a simple, uncomplicated life is also really important to me. But I am able to create financial security and abundance for myself and my family. And I absolutely love my job and my work and my patients, and feel so grateful every day.

I'm passionate about helping other acupuncturists do and feel the same. I have been teaching business and marketing to acupuncturists since 2012. I've led classes at CSTCM and SWAC, webinars, online courses, and coaching programs. I've built my own practice, trained and mentored several associates, coached many other acupuncturists, and I've seen time and time again how powerful this information can be.

I didn't get into this field because I was interested in learning about marketing or running my own business, so if marketing and business don't excite you, that's ok. I got into it because I experienced its healing power first hand, and wanted to bring this amazing medicine to more people. I chose to go to acupuncture school because I wanted to help people while having a career that was meaningful to me. I was deeply unsatisfied in my previous career in finance. I wanted my work to make the world a better place and leave a positive impact on people. I thought I'd leave my job as a financial analyst to do development work giving micro loans to women in developing countries, and spent months in India volunteering and studying yoga and Vedanta philosophy. When I had health issues of my own, and doctors didn't have any answers, I tried acupuncture and was blown away. I knew I'd found my calling. I immediately enrolled in acupuncture school.

My desire was to spend my working hours connecting with people on a deep level (rather than staring at spreadsheets) which felt like a natural gift and proclivity of mine, to feel my work made the world a better place, and more specifically to support women in a meaningful way. Being an acupuncturist fit this perfectly. As a finance person, I did some quick math in my head: My acupuncturist charged $65 per visit. Multiply that by forty hours a week. That's $135,200 a year in revenue. But, I would need the patients to fill those spots. That turned out to be the hard part.

I thought that my commitment to helping people and the results of my services would be enough to propel my practice. I envisioned people lining up outside my door, eager for my help. What actually happened is that I opened my practice, printed business cards, slapped up a website, and then… crickets. I was freaked. I had a small fortune in student loan debt from grad school. I HAD to make this work.

So, I began marketing. I designed, printed and hand-delivered one thousand flyers in the neighborhood around my clinic, thinking people just needed to know that I was there and eager to help. This resulted in more crickets. I was devastated. I had left my job and dedicated years of schooling to honing a skill that I knew could benefit so many people. That was the most frustrating part – knowing that so many people needed acupuncture and TCM, but not knowing how to convince them.

That's when I had an "aha" moment: I knew absolutely nothing about marketing. Loving my medicine didn't mean I had any clue how to sell it. I realized that if I was committed to my medicine and my practice, I'd have to become my own marketing team.

I read as many marketing books as I could find, and, to my surprise, learned that good marketing is soulful and authentic, and it requires empathy, connection, and compassion. I started experimenting and implementing these newly learned strategies in my clinic. I found some marketing advice to be ineffective in our industry, and other techniques to be especially potent. I developed a clear understanding of who I wanted to work with and why. I tweaked my website for search engine optimization, I blogged, and I designed another more specific and benefit-driven flyer for my neighborhood. My efforts resulted in twenty-one new patients from the flyers alone. Not bad!! In months, I was consistently seeing thirty patients per week. The following year, I was hovering around forty-five patients per week, which I felt was my max capacity if I also wanted to keep my sanity. After my student loans were paid off, I set limits to the hours I worked, started a waiting list, and hired associates.

Did the surge in business make everything easier? Well, no. I was working double time to run my practice, treat patients, and keep my marketing fresh on top of that. I put so much energy into trying everything I was learning about marketing (including things that didn't work), and I was getting burnt out. I remember thinking to myself: if only someone could have shown me the ropes – which marketing strategies work effectively for an acupuncture clinic. Even with my newfound success, I spent those first three years feeling overwhelmed, anxious, and frustrated.

Did I get through it and build a profitable and sustainable practice that I love? Yes. Could the process have been more efficient and joyful? Yes. That's why I'm so passionate about helping other acupuncturists in their practices. I've been there, I know how hard and anxiety-provoking it is. I want to show you that you can do it, and it doesn't need to be so hard.

Too many acupuncturists are struggling to fill their schedule, worrying about money, relying on a part-time job to support themselves, and not helping the number of people they'd like to be. The solution, I believe, is better marketing – the skill of communicating what you do and how it helps people.

I cringe inside when I hear acupuncturists say, "All you need to build a successful practice are results, results, results." It plays to our insecurities, and it's inaccurate. Being a great acupuncturist alone isn't enough to get the success you deserve.

Don't let anyone make you feel like you aren't already well-prepared to give great acupuncture treatments. You received an excellent education and clinical training and I'd wager to say you already get great results and that if you don't, if you simply got your patients in more frequently for treatment you'd get great results. The common statement that all you need is results is not only patronizing and preys on our insecurities, but it has the potential to distract us from focusing on another important piece necessary for success. You need results AND you need to understand and embrace marketing.

Taking continuing education classes and honing your treatment skills will absolutely benefit your practice, your patients, and help your confidence. But it isn't *everything* you'll need for business success. Because here's the thing to remember: it takes time to get those results; on average, it takes eight to ten treatments for a patient to get dramatic results (based on a survey of over 200 acupuncturists and various conditions). This means you must communicate with your patients so that they'll come back as many times as it takes to achieve those great results, communicating and marketing in a way that inspires confidence and trust. It's all about intentional, strategic, authentic communication as well as good results. When you combine marketing know-how with your skilled treatments, passion and authentic voice, you will become unstoppable.

In this book, I'm going to show you how to:

- Build a business that's in line with you and your values
- Retain patients authentically
- Articulate your message so that it resonates with the people you most want to serve

- Create a marketing plan that's in alignment with who you are and attracts patients on autopilot
- Overcome your inner critic and limiting beliefs
- And more

These skills are the Jing behind a successful clinic. You simply can't prosper without them. And the world needs you to prosper. You can do it, my friend.

we have to hold on
to the big because

Chapter 1

Bring your vision Into Focus

Society is constantly nudging us to chase our dreams. But before you start anything, it's wise to define your goals and your "why". Create a vision. Otherwise, you're doomed to accept the status quo.

I'm not here to accept the status quo. The world has its problems, and we acupuncturists have the answers to many of those problems. Here's my vision.

I want to live in a world where...

Acupuncture and Chinese medicine are well-regarded, widely used, respected and lucrative professions that are considered part of the standard care domain...

A mother's first instinct is to get shonishin and herbs for her child, not antibiotics, when her child has come down with an ear infection or cough...

People go to the ER to get a bone reset and sutures put in, but then decline the pain medications and opt to go to their acupuncturist to promote true healing after an injury…

Women routinely visit their acupuncturists before trying to conceive to prepare their bodies for optimal fertility…

People know that a diagnosis of "IBS" or "chronic fatigue" is not a life sentence, and that a root problem can be addressed to heal their bodies…

It's common knowledge that insomnia or indigestion are not symptoms to be suppressed, but calls for help to be heeded and addressed…

Many acupuncturists struggle to grow their practices because they haven't been taught the business fundamentals that are necessary to sustain a practice without burning out. And that makes me so sad.

I want you to have the skills and know-how to make your practice work for you without being overwhelming, and reach the patients that need you so.

I want the world to know that acupuncture is a no-brainer and first line of defense, rather than a last-ditch effort to be undertaken skeptically after all other avenues have been tried.

I believe the world will be a better place when we have more compassionate, CONFIDENT, and business-savvy acupuncturists who step into their power, build strong brands, expand their practice to reach a greater audience, and show the world that we mean business.

That's my why and my vision, what's yours?

"Never doubt that a small group of thoughtful, committed, citizens can change the world, indeed, it is the only thing that ever has."

— Margaret Mead

Bring your vision into focus and create a meaningful future

What are your heart and soul urging you to do, even if it scares you? You don't need to have it all figured out; you just need to start bringing your vision into focus. In the words of Abraham Hicks, "Use your imagination until your big dream feels so familiar that the manifestation is the next logical step."

Studies such as *Psychology Today's* "Seeing is Believing," published in 2009, demonstrate how powerful visualization can be in shaping future outcomes and prove that thoughts produce the same mental structures as actions. Thanks to neuroplasticity (the ability of the brain to continuously create new neural pathways), when we repeat a task, we strengthen the neural networks needed to perform it. The same thing happens in our brains whether we perform the action or just visualize it.

So harness this and use it to your advantage by making time to visualize what you want. When you use your mind to cultivate stories of what you want (rather than what you don't want) and really feel the feeling of what you want to create, wonderful things can happen for you.

your brain literally can't tell the difference between the actions you perform and the actions you visualized.

Here's an exercise to help you lean into powerful visualization:

1. Identify the outcome you desire.
2. Visualize the outcome until it's as though it's happening now. What do you see? What do you feel? What do you hear?
3. Expand on that feeling. Make the image bigger. Relish in it, like it's really happening.

Talk yourself into your dreams,
not out of them

"When you want something,
all the universe conspires
in helping you to achieve it."

— Paulo Coelho

Chapter 2

The World Needs Us Now More Than Ever

Is there a demand for acupuncture? A resounding yes! Let's look at some statistics:

Chronic disease, pain, and mental health issues are on the rise. According to the CDC, six in ten adults have a chronic disease, and one in four have multiple conditions.

The prevalence for all of these are expected to rise. The rate of chronic disease in kids more than doubled between 1994 and 2006. Rates of autoimmune disease have tripled over the past 50 years, and are expected to continue to rise sharply.

Acupuncture and Asian Medicine can help. This is where we acupuncturists shine. Western medicine is amazing for acute emergencies, injuries, and infections. But when it comes to chronic diseases like autoimmune disease, IBS, and fibromyalgia, it falls short. When it comes to pain, it falls short and leads to addiction and side effects. When it comes to mental health like anxiety and depression, it falls short. Many patients of chronic pain find that their prescribed Western treatments help very little, if at all. They accept these things as lifelong conditions without considering alternatives.

More and more people are turning to acupuncture, but it's still not enough. According to NHIS survey data, acupuncture usage in America has increased significantly, rising from 4.2% of the population (8.19 million) to 6.3% (12.01 million) between 2002 and 2007. That's a 47% increase in acupuncture usage in 5 years, a trend that is expected to continue. And acupuncture usage has an even greater prevalence worldwide.

Studies show that patients are loving acupuncture. An independent study of 89,000 acupuncture patients treated in 2014 and 2015 found high rates of satisfaction, exceeding national benchmarks' averages. Up to 93% of those surveyed said their acupuncturist succeeded in addressing their primary health issue. Up to 87% of survey responders rated their acupuncturists at a 9 or a 10 on a ten-point scale. The national averages for conventional care providers for those years were between 76%-80%. Many of these patients had stubborn, chronic pain conditions that weren't relieved by conventional treatment. To see such high satisfaction rates in that demographic is really remarkable.

But the health and outcome statistics are only part of the story of why patients need us. Many patients are disappointed and frustrated with the care they're getting from Western doctors. Without getting real solutions, they don't feel listened to or treated with dignity. They're frustrated with being told they're "fine" when they're suffering, and with endless testing that doesn't lead to deeper understanding. They're prescribed medications that don't actually heal the problem, and only lead to more side effects. What they want is to be listened to, spoken to respectfully, educated about their choices, and given clear options (and clear costs) for solutions. They want to be empowered to participate in their own care, and to actually heal and thrive. This is exactly what acupuncturists can give them.

We acupuncturists also give people what they crave on a deeper level, too. I believe people these days are hungry for meaning, self-understanding, and connection. We live in a rushed, digital, disconnected time. People are overwhelmed with all the information constantly bombarding them. Our attention spans have gotten shorter, and people are more distracted and isolated.

In our acupuncture clinics, part of our role is to create a space where patients are really heard; where they matter. You may be the first one to listen to and validate your patient in their healing journey. With your help, they'll gain a deeper understanding of themselves and their symptoms. And they'll also get in touch with themselves as they're forced to spend 30 minutes in a quiet, phone-free zone. This creation of order, understanding, meaning, and connection is something that soothes people on a deep level.

It's a great time to be an acupuncturist. The demand for our services is there. People need us now more than ever.

Deep down you know exactly what you're capable of.

Chapter 3

So why are so many acupuncturists struggling?

So the demand is there and the world needs us, yet so many acupuncturists are struggling.

Surveys have shown that the majority of acupuncturists are earning a gross income of $20-60,000 a year. After taxes, student loans and living expenses, that's a net balance of only $10-30,000 annually for the majority of acupuncturists. On top of this, a survey from 2009 showed that most acupuncturists averaged $87,000 in student loan debt. Yikes. Acupuncturists are not making enough money, or similarly, impacting the number of lives they could be!

Our medicine is amazing; patients should be flocking to you, and your business should be booming! So, why are acupuncturists barely surviving when they should be thriving?

Well, I think it's pretty clear how we got here: lack of business education and a cultural mindset within our schools and profession that disdains business. One practice management class in your last semester is NOT enough to set you up for success, especially if you have a mindset that you're either above business or doomed to struggle. Our education puts us TENS of THOUSANDS of dollars into debt. We're shoved into the world hoping that we will succeed. But, as I've just cited above, most acupuncturists are taking home less than $30,000 a year! But it doesn't have to be this way, and I'm hoping this book will help in a meaningful way.

visualize your highest self and start showing up as her

Chapter 4

What's Possible for you

Empowered acupuncturists can change the world and make a good living while doing it. And that's exactly why I created AcuProsper.

Some encouraging ~~words~~ math

Here's some math that I think is important and inspiring to understand, so even though it's dry, please follow me on a little math equation. Let's assume the rent for a two-room clinic is $1,000 a month. The cost of needles, alcohol, and supplies is about $100 a month. Wi-Fi, website hosting, and EHR software are another $200 a month. CEUs are $100 a month. Malpractice insurance is another $100 a month. And then, let's round up another $500 for miscellaneous expenses. This brings business costs to about $2000 a month. This accurately reflects what my costs are, by the way.

Ok, now let's assume your price per treatment is $75 on average. Let's also assume a 30% tax rate on profits, and 2 weeks of vacation a year.

With these assumptions, how much would you be able to pay yourself in take-home pay a year if you saw…

- 10 patients/week = $13,500 (pre-tax) ➔ $9,450 (after tax)
- 15 patients/week = $32,250   ➔ $22,575
- 20 patients/week = $51,000   ➔ $35,700
- 25 patients/week = $69,750   ➔ $48,825
- 30 patients/week = $88,500   ➔ $61,950
- 35 patients/week = $107,250   ➔ $75,075
- 40 patients/week = $126,000   ➔ $88,200
- 45 patients/week = $144,750   ➔ $101,325
- 50 patients/week = $163,500   ➔ $114,450

You'll probably need a receptionist and more than two treatment rooms after that point, which will increase your costs and change our assumptions and equation, so let's stop at 50 patients a week, even though more is certainly possible.

This math illustrates two important points: 1) why acupuncturists can barely make ends meet and feel so doomed when they're seeing 10 – 20 patients a week; 2) that you can make a good living once you're above a certain threshold of patient visits per week. Looking at the math in this example, once acupuncturists get above 30 or so patients a week, because their overhead is the same as before (rent, etc.) and their marginal costs have hardly increased (needles and cotton balls are pennies extra per patient), their income level increases significantly. An increase of just ten patients per week makes a huge difference in income.

Would earning $144,750 in take-home pay seeing 45 patients a week allow you to pay off your student loans in a few years and live a good life? I'd say so. All while improving lives and doing what you love. How awesome is that? You just have to get to that number of patient volume, which is totally doable (and which you can see in less than 40 hours of work a week if you have more than one treatment room). The take-home here is that you can indeed make a good living as an acupuncturist without working yourself to the bone, and that marketing is key since patient numbers are key.

you often feel tired,
not because you've done
too much, but because you've
done too little of what
lights a fire inside you.

Determining your values and what success means to you

The word "success" makes me cringe a little because… what does it *mean,* really? Personally, I'm partial to the quote, "Inner peace is the new success." Heck yeah! That little sentence packs a punch. To me, inner peace is feeling good about my work. It's feeling like I'm contributing to making the world a better place; feeling like the way I spend my time and energy is in alignment with who I am, my natural gifts, and my values; feeling both challenged and supported towards growth and self-improvement; and not worrying about finances, knowing that myself and my family will have enough now and in the future. That's what both inner peace and success mean to me. But I think it means different things to everyone. What does it mean to you?

Here's what I emphasize to my Clinical Practice Management students on the very first day of class: Determine your values so that you can design your practice so that it supports your values and highest priorities. The way to do this is to take a look at where your energy, time, money, emotions, and inner and outer dialogue go. As I learned from the author John Demartini, our life reflects what's true in our hearts, what we care about and what's important to us. Always.

Where are you most organized in life? What do you find yourself externally dialoging about, and when the conversation hits a lull, what do you bring up? Look around your home. What do you physically fill your space with - what do you see? Do you see a guitar, a stack of recipe books, your ski equipment, or photos of your family? When you have extra cash, what do you spend it on? When you have extra time outside of work, how do you spend it? Do you spend it in nature, with friends or family, on your health, on self-growth, travelling, studying, shopping, cooking…? The answers to these questions can point you toward what your values and priorities are.

For example, when answering those questions, it became clear that eating and preparing healthy food is a high value of mine. I should have known, then, that when I was busting my rear to grow my practice and pay off my student loans, working until 7pm five days a week, that I'd get burnt out and resentful. Why? Not because I was working *too much*, but because of what I *wasn't doing*. I wasn't making it home in time to cook myself a good dinner. I was scarfing down cold leftovers whenever I got a free second at the clinic. Now, for someone else, that probably wouldn't be a big deal. But for me, over time, it really wore on me, and even though my clinic was thriving, I felt deflated. I think we often feel burnt out and frustrated not because we're doing too much, but because we're doing too little of what lights a fire inside of us. If I had simply set my schedule to honor my values - so that I could at least make it home in time to cook a healthy meal a couple times a week - I would have been happier. And it's best to know this from the beginning, although it's never too late to readjust.

Success starts with your vision, and more specifically, a vision that honors and supports your highest values. You don't have to create a business that looks just like your mentor's or anyone else's, instead create one that serves the life you want to lead. I encourage you to explore and honor what your values are, and to set up your business so that it's in alignment with your particular value hierarchy. You might need to get creative. If travel is a high value of yours, for example, make sure that either your rent is low so it's not a big deal to take a whole month off to travel or plan to hire associates so they can cover you while you're gone. If you want to make sure you have time to exercise or eat, honor that and make it happen for yourself. Otherwise, that "inner peace" doesn't come easily, regardless of how many patients you're seeing or money you're making. Income does not directly translate to "success," in my opinion. However, we are constantly converting our income into our highest values by deciding what to do with it. So, if we have enough disposable income to help us fulfill and support our highest values, I think that can contribute to a feeling of inner peace and happiness, which to me is what I'd call "success." Meaning that success is individual to each of us.

What helped me:

Take time to observe and notice what your life has taught you in terms of what you value most highly. Answer these questions:

Where do you spend your extra money? Where are you most organized? What do you externally dialogue about most? What do you internally dialogue around and set goals toward most? What do you physically fill your space with? How do you spend your free time?

Write down the answers, then go back and count the number of times something was repeated. The things repeated the most? Those are your highest values, my friend. Circle them. Honor them.

_____

_____

_____

_____

_____

_____

Having a specific goal based on numbers was very empowering for me. It helped me to stay focused, measure my progress, and celebrate my wins and growth along the way.

Exercise: Use math to figure out your goal number of patient visits per week.

1. What pre-tax monthly income would you like to pay yourself? _____

2. What are your total monthly business expenses? (always round up to be conservative) _____

3. Add those two lines. That's the monthly revenue you need to make _____

4. Now multiply the above # by 12 to get an annual revenue figure _____

5. How many weeks of vacation would you like to take? Use that to figure out how many weeks a year you would like to work. (There are 52 weeks in a year, so subtract the # of weeks of vacation you'd like to take from 52)

   _____

6. Divide the # in 4 by the # in 5. That's how much revenue you need to make per working week

   _____

7. What's your average price per visit? _____

8. Divide #6 by #7. This is the # of patient visits you need a week in order to bring home your goal income

   _____

** I recommend you return to line 1, increase the monthly income you'd like to pay yourself, and do the exercise again. I'm guessing you low-balled yourself the first time to fit what you think is possible. I want you to aim a little higher, my friend, because you can do it.

What I really want you to see is what's possible. Clearly, you CAN make a generous income as an acupuncturist. And you can do it in LESS than 40 hours a week if you're treating out of two or more rooms, which means that you can hopefully make time and space for your other priorities and values. Even better? You can feel GREAT about what you do, about your life's work. You're improving lives. You're changing the world. That. Is. Awesome.

So please don't give up. Please dream big. Please don't get stuck in small thinking, such as never expecting to be able to earn enough to buy a house or pay off your student loans. Because the demand is there for your services. You just need to let them know that you're there and available to help them, and that's what I'll show you how to do.

Chapter 5

Bridging the Gap

So, the world needs us, but most acupuncturists are struggling. What gives? How do we bridge this gap between huge consumer need and low business profits for acupuncturists?

In a perfect world, we acupuncturists would all band together and fund a public health campaign along the lines of the famous "Got milk?" and "click it or ticket" campaigns. I would call it the "diet, lifestyle, and acupuncture first" campaign.

But until that day comes, each of us is in charge of our own PR. Granted, a rising tide lifts all boats. So, when one of us acupuncturists does a great job in educating people about the benefits of acupuncture, it helps the rest of us, too.

But you can't sit back and let others do your work for you. We've each got to take the bull by the horns and let the world know that we're here, and that we can help. We've got to show people exactly how we can help them.

Now, while there is no such thing as a magical pill, there is one skill that has fueled the success that I'm grateful to have today: communicating my value with confidence. This is what makes people want to work with you, and commit to the treatment plan you lay out.

In the past, jobs were about muscle, now they're about brains, but in the future they'll be about hearts."

— Minouche Shafik, director,
London School of Economics

It doesn't matter how great of an acupuncturist or herbalist you are if no one knows about you, trusts you, or gets you. That's what marketing is – letting people know about you and how you can help them while cultivating their trust in you. And it's your responsibility to make this happen. Let this be your wake-up call, because I know that so many of us resist this reality. If you have a service that makes the world a better place (which you do), then it is your responsibility to let the world know about it. It's your responsibility to let people know that you're there and that you can help them, and to explain how your services will improve their lives.

I heard a story about Tony Robbins talking to a woman during one if his events. He asked her what she did for work, and she told him she's a postpartum doula. She helps women during one of the most transformative periods of their life to reclaim their power, and to heal and rest and recover and feel their best. She loves what she does, and her clients love her too. Tony then asked her how she gets new clients, and she told him, "Oh, I'm really bad about marketing and getting new clients in." What Tony said shocked me. He replied, "Oh, so you suck at what you do."

I saw this as an attack on this doula's valuable profession, thinking she should instead be lauded for her work. But he went on to say that getting clients in is just as much a part of her job as supporting them postpartum. He said that she can't transform their lives unless she gets them to sign up - that's just half of her job.

I resisted it and resented it at first, but he had a point that makes sense. A point that, unfortunately, defines our reality, too. Even if you have the solution to the world's problems, that won't do any good if you can't figure out how to tell them. And that is, in fact, part of your job.

Many acupuncturists resist this because they are under the misconception that marketing is pushy or salesy. Let me ask you something: Do you like listening to people and trying to figure out what they need? Do you like to help people solve problems and lead healthier, happier lives? Do you like talking about things that you are passionate about? Do you like inspiring people to action and helping them live up to their full potential? If you said yes to any of that, I've got news for you: You already love marketing!

Now, here's the part that can really surprise you. When you do this well, the best and most loving parts of you come out, because to be fully effective, you must listen fully, deeply and openly; you must be compassionate enough to really understand how your patient feels, what they need, what they fear, what they dream of. You need to come from a place of love, because people can feel whether you really care. Good marketing isn't pushy or salesy, it's soulful and requires empathy and compassion.

Once you really get this kind of marketing, you're going to be able to let the people who most need you know that you're there, that you can help them, and that they need you. You'll be able to make your services a no-brainer for them. You'll be able to make more money, and more importantly, help more patients.

If we acupuncturists collectively embrace this, we'll be able to elevate our profession, change public opinion about acupuncture, educate the public about the amazing benefits and results of our care, and make the world a better place. This, I believe, is how we bridge the gap, and if you try on this perspective, it will transform your business and your life.

your softness is the strongest
and most powerful part of you.

Chapter 6

Key Mindset

So, where do we start? I think that our mindset is just the place.

The first step is embracing the above paradigm shift about marketing and communicating our value.

What comes next?

Think win-win

The number one mindset for success and fulfillment in business is a win-win attitude, meaning that you make sure that with your services, you win, the patient wins, the world wins - everyone wins.

Win-lose thinking comes from the belief that the success of others will mean less success for you; or that your success will mean that someone else has to lose. This will only lead to resentment, shame, or burnout, and going out of business (ultimately meaning that the patients lose too).

"what if I fall?
Oh, but my darling,
what if you fly?"

— Erin Hansen

Win-win thinking:

- Charge a fair price (and don't give discounts beyond your listed and customary discounts)
- Stick to your listed hours, and don't work hours that will leave you burned out or resentful
- Run on time and don't add on unnecessary services that deplete you and leave you burned out or resentful
- Respectfully and compassionately stick to your principles, and advise your patients in their best interests in terms of treatment frequency and lifestyle recommendations.

To think win-win, you need to champion the other person's "win" as much as your own. The key is that *everyone wins*. You get to practice this amazing medicine that you love, you get to support yourself and your family, your healed patients can live more fulfilled lives, and the world is a better place. Everyone wins.

This attitude creates gratitude, appreciation, and good vibes, and it magnetically attracts more of the same. When you feel this, I believe the universe sends you more opportunities to create this good will, which leads to growth.

If you are thinking that you've got to lose, that you have to work too much and get paid too little in order for other people to win, I don't think that you're going to be successful. I don't think that the universe will send you more patients if you only feel resentment and anger every time you swipe someone's credit card because you're charging them too little. I don't think that's the recipe for success and attracting more to you.

And similarly, if you feel shame or guilt because you feel like you're overcharging someone or making them pay a big premium upfront while assuming all the risk, I don't believe the universe is going to send you more opportunities to continue this exploitation.

I think that when you feel appreciation and gratitude, and you think, "I'm winning, you're winning, everyone's winning, and this is great. I get to help you, and I get to do what I love, and pay off my student loans, and support my family," that is the recipe for success.

It's got to be mutually beneficial and win-win. If you're interested in reading more about this, a great book all about this is *The Go Giver* - I highly recommend it. Watch out for others' interests, not just your own. Focus on the other person's win. I scratched your back, now you owe me - that's not being a friend, that's being a creditor. Stop keeping score. Which leads us to the next item...

Contribution

Another key mindset for practice success is to make it about what you can give versus what you can get. Focus first on what you can contribute to your customers, to society, to your team, and to the people you love; this will attract people and opportunities to you, and you will be rewarded.

The majority of people operate with a mindset that says to the fireplace, "First, give me some heat, then I'll throw on some logs." And of course, it doesn't work that way. Successful people keep their focus on what they're giving, sharing, etc. When people focus on contributing, on adding value, on practicing outflowing, they become irresistible, and their businesses become irresistible. How do you serve and give value to others? That should be your first question.

"We have to keep walking our own path, keep writing our own story, and trust that somehow it will all unfold in the right way"

— Unknown

Some of my favorite ways of doing this are: 1) Answering peoples' questions when they call or email to ask if acupuncture could help their specific situation, rather than telling them to just schedule an appointment and you'll talk about it then. I've heard from so many patients over the years that I was the only one who took the time to talk to them over the phone or email, and that's why they chose to come to me. 2) Sharing your wisdom via blogging, videos, giving talks, or social media. If you aim to contribute to peoples' lives a little bit for free, without them having to come pay you for an acupuncture session, your life and practice will be overflowing.

It's how the universe works – you've got to put logs on the fire first, and then you'll feel the warmth. Don't be a martyr and give away your services without equitable exchange (money, referrals, trust, experience, etc.), but absolutely aim to make peoples' lives better by answering their questions and sharing a bit of your vast knowledge.

Imagine that there are two acupuncturists. They are both very experienced and gifted Chinese medicine practitioners. Acupuncturist A believes potential patients must pay for his services in order to benefit from his knowledge. He sees blogging as giving away his knowledge for free and devaluing what he does. When people call his office, he says, "come in for an appointment and we can talk about your condition." He feels put out and imposed upon by championing their wins without getting paid first.

Acupuncturist B blogs about her medicine, answers specific questions generously on social media and for free, chats with potential patients about their condition on the phone when they call to enquire about services, and refers to other practitioners when she thinks it might help a patient.

Who do you think has more patients clamoring for their services? The person who has contributed more and championed others' wins. Why? Potential clients have gotten a taste for Acupuncturist B's approach, philosophy, ability and willingness to help, whereas it feels like a bigger leap of faith to trust Acupuncturist A because he hasn't given a taste for what he can do. Acupuncturist B's generosity and openness has lowered the perceived risk and uncertainty, and it's easy to see how she can help you. Acupuncturist B's method ultimately leads to rewards. When practitioners are willing to share their talents, inspirations, and gifts with the world, the rewards they receive in return will be even more abundant.

What are your talents? What are you good at? Acknowledge it and give it away. What can I do today instead of what can today do for me? The Greek philosophy, "Know yourself, control yourself, give yourself." is very wise.

Of course, you don't need to be a martyr and lose in order for others to win. Maintain good boundaries, charge a fair price, touch peoples' lives. Your healing work deserves to be supported; you deserve to be paid fairly. But the key is to focus on contributing value to the world.

If you start to feel resentment or burnout, that's a sign that you're giving too much of yourself away without fair compensation or appreciation, and that perhaps you are edging to a lose-win mentality. So, tune into that, but don't expect people to appreciate your value, sign up to work with you, pay you, or refer friends to you BEFORE you've shared your value or contributed to the betterment of their lives in some way.

Show up for your dreams

Chapter 7

Too Legit to Quit

The next step to showing the world, and yourself, that you mean business is to set up a legitimate and well-structured business.

In the United States, it's incredibly easy, fast, and inexpensive to start a business. In Colorado, for instance, fifty bucks and thirty minutes is all it takes to have an officially registered LLC or S-Corp. How amazing is that?

You don't even necessarily need a lawyer, as the Secretary of State website walks you through creating your very own Articles of Organization. If you have specific questions or unique circumstances, absolutely hire a lawyer to help you. But it's a nice bonus that hiring a lawyer isn't absolutely necessary.

Do your research and understand the differences between Sole Proprietor, LLC, and S-Corps, and which one is the best fit for you, your situation, your goals and your state. There are legal and tax implications that you should understand. Your business class in acupuncture school should have helped you with this, so hopefully, you have this all dialed in. If not, then my course, "Start Your Acupuncture Clinic," is a good resource for you. As is this free mini-course: https://acuprosper.thinkific.com/courses/business-models. If you're still not sure, then I recommend hiring an accountant and/or lawyer to help you. Don't worry, it's not too late to get this in place if you don't yet feel good about your current structure - you can change your business structure with the help of an accountant and/or lawyer even if you've been in practice for years already. But absolutely make sure you feel good about the structure and legitimacy of your business, and don't let any fears around that hold you back.

You want to feel a sense of confidence, trust, and security knowing that all your ducks are in a row, and that you have all the necessary paperwork, and that you're legally protected. You want to have all the proper systems in place. A fear or uncertainty over the legitimacy of your business can subconsciously keep you playing small and limit your success. You want to be open to being a smashing success, because you know you are legit. This subconsciously sends a message to yourself about what's possible, and it sends a message to the world, too – you mean business.

Finances and getting started

If you want to succeed, you absolutely need a financial plan. Specifically, if you're just starting out, you need to have an idea of:

1. What it will cost you to get started (if you're not already up and running)
2. Your monthly business expenses
3. How many patient visits it will take to cover those monthly expenses
4. How much you need to pay yourself in order to support your lifestyle and pay off your student loans
5. How many patient visits per month it will take to do that (adding this to the # of patient visits from line (3)

6. An estimate of how long it will take to get to that point of seeing your goal # of patient visits a month, and

7. A plan for how you will cover yourself until you do get to that point.

Every one of our clinics will be unique, so I recommend doing this exercise and calculations for your own unique vision and situation. For example, some of us will have multiple rooms, some won't have a waiting room they need to furnish, and so on. Close your eyes, imagine your clinic in the mental gallery of your mind, and imagine walking through it room by room – what do you see? Make a wish list, and then make estimates on what you think it will cost to procure those things. In case it's helpful, here are some example start-up costs (pulled from a spreadsheet I share in the How to Start Your Acupuncture Clinic course based on my own personal experience and budget):

- Rent deposit - $800
- Internet - $60
- Board exams/License - $1000
- Web hosting (annual) - $70
- Quickbooks software - $300
- Printer/scanner - $100
- Waiting room chairs - $180
- Waiting room side table - $50
- Tablet or computer - $500
- Waiting room décor - $100
- Reception desk - $200
- Reception chair - $50

- Water dispenser and cups - $50
- Treatment room side table - $90
- Treatment room shelf/cabinet - $100
- Treatment room desk - $150
- Desk chair - $60
- Patient intake chair - $90
- Treatment room décor - $100
- Heat lamp - $200
- Massage table - $200
- Sheets and blankets - $150
- Pillows and bolsters - $40
- Needles - $150
- Cups - $40
- Cotton balls and alcohol - $15
- Sharps containers plus mail-back service - $90
- Paper, clipboards, pens, Kleenex, cleaning products - $100
- Office signage - $100
- Business cards - $100

This comes to a total start-up cost of $5,249. While that can feel like a lot when you're just graduating from school with no income coming in and a high uncertainty level about going it alone, think of it as the cost of starting a BUSINESS and empowering yourself to touch lives and do what you love. With that perspective, it's not much in the scheme of things, and we are so lucky that the equipment necessary to be in practice is so minimal.

Estimating your start-up costs is something that your business class in acupuncture school hopefully covered, but if not, now's your chance. If you're already established and in practice, but you have dreams of moving or creating a different clinic someday, you can use this exercise to get an idea of what the start-up costs would be for your dream clinic:

Step 1: close your eyes and imagine your clinic - what do you see?

Step 2: write down your wish list for your clinic

Step 3: write down your equipment wish list for your clinic

Step 4: research the costs of the above two steps and write it down. You can make two lists – a "Dream Big" list and a "Start Small" list – if you like.

Step 5: look around for office spaces that would work for you and your vision (perhaps on Craiglist). Find the location, size, and vibe that would work for you. Get an idea of what that would cost. Write it down. (This will likely be both a start-up cost because of a first and last month's rent deposit as well as a monthly recurring cost.)

Add them up and these are your start-up costs.

If you look at your wish-list start-up cost forecast, and it's more than you feel you can afford, remember: You can tweak it so it's right for your unique situation. You could start smaller and grow into your vision over time. Starting small does not mean playing small. For example, you could rent an already furnished room in another clinic, thereby saving yourself the start-up investment in furniture and decreasing your rent. But it's a great idea to have this wish-list start-up cost estimate based on your vision that you're working toward. That way, you'll know how much to save up before you start looking for your own space and take that leap towards your vision.

Other than education cost, it doesn't *have* to cost much to start your clinic. Of course, it *could* cost a lot, but it doesn't *have* to. It depends on your vision and plan. On a related side note, I think that it's wise to view your student loans as a start-up cost. While that huge pile of debt may give you heart palpitations, realize that your education is a business investment; you couldn't start a clinic or be in business without it. When I realized this for myself, it made me feel much more grateful and empowered. Investing $100,000 to start a business? That's actually nothing compared to a lot of businesses!

Next, you need to know how much it will cost to run your clinic on a monthly basis. Here are example monthly expenses, pulled from a spreadsheet in my How to Start Your Acupuncture Clinic course and from my own clinic, in case it's helpful for you:

- Rent - $800
- Liability insurance - $41.67 ($500 a year in your first year of practice)
- Cell phone - $90
- Personal health insurance - $265
- Continuing education - $100
- EHR and online scheduling - $60
- Misc. office supplies (paper, ink, Kleenex, pens) - $40
- Water and cups - $30
- License and professional association memberships - $15
- Accountant - $20.83 ($250 a year)
- Needles - $75

- Cotton balls, alcohol - $5
- Sharps container service - $30

This adds up to a total monthly business expense of $1,612. You can see that rent is the bulk of that (so, just a reminder to be smart with the space you choose, which we'll talk about in a bit). I recommend dividing that number by your average treatment price (and by the way, I give you a pre-formatted spreadsheet for these calculations in the AcuProsper How to Start Your Clinic course, in case the math is overwhelming for you). Let's say your average treatment price is $75. $1,612 divided by $75 is 21.5. That means you'd need to see about 22 patients a month, or 5.5 a week, in order to cover your expenses. That's really important to know!

Next, think about how much you'd like to take home a month in income before tax. Let's say it's $5,000. Divide that number by your average treatment price. In this example, $5,000 divided by $75 is 67. Add that number to the number we previously calculated (to determine the minimum patient load to cover expenses). In this example, that's 67 + 22, so you'd have to see 89 patients a month, or about 22 a week in order to cover your costs and pay yourself $5,000 a month.

That's powerful, to have the clarity of that specific goal in your mind! Twenty-two patients a week is totally doable! I recommend going back and increasing that take-home pay. Dream big, and do that calculation again. Set high goals, and know that it's totally doable! The real beauty in our profession is that your income is directly tied to the number of people you HELP and serve. You should feel good about it. Your healing work deserves to be lovingly supported and rewarded and honored and appreciated - don't forget that.

But here's an important thing to keep in mind and plan for: If you're just starting out, it will take time to get to that goal (in this example, twenty-two patients a week). I recommend estimating as best you can – how long do you think it will take you to get there? Everyone's situation is going to be different; this is where openness among acupuncturists is beneficial. It can be helpful to talk to friends and hear about their experiences with clinic growth. I'm happy to be open about my experience. I hit 20 patients a week after 10 months. I saw 5 patients a week from the very first week I was in business (I moved to Denver to open my clinic and knew hardly anyone), so from day one of opening my clinic doors, I was profitable and not losing money – which is rare in business! Again, yay for our low overhead costs! But I wasn't able to take home $5,000 a month for quite some time. The question then is, what's the plan for supporting yourself until you hit that goal?

For this, I recommend asking yourself, what's the *minimum* you need to take home in order to survive? Look at your personal expenses – what do you absolutely need to take home? At the time when I was starting my clinic, I needed to take home $1500 (I was single, living with roommates, and keeping a tight budget). Once you have your minimum number, calculate how many patients you would need to see a week in order to meet that. In my example, $1500 divided by $75 is 20 patient visits a month, or 5 patient visits a week. Add that to the number of patient visits needed to cover my business expenses, which was 5.5 in the example above - so 5.5 + 5 = 10.5 patient visits a week in order to cover my expenses and pay myself enough to get by. The next question to ask is, how long do you think it will take to hit that goal? I was seeing 10 patients a week within three months of opening my clinic. That meant that I needed to have enough money saved up to support myself without a salary for three months, until I was seeing enough patients to be able to pay myself enough to live on. Luckily, I had done these calculations in school while planning my business, and I had enough saved up to support myself for six months while I grew my business. I realize that not all of us are fortunate to have savings, so the important thing to ask yourself is, what's my plan for paying myself while I grow? Will I get a part-time job? Will I apply for a loan? Borrow from family? This is where that saying comes in "if you fail to plan, you plan to fail." Don't give up and go out of business because you couldn't support yourself in those crucial first few months. Make a plan for how you'll make it while you're growing. Knowing that math can be extremely empowering. There are three goals I recommend you know:

- The number of patient visits a week you need to cover your business expenses _____

- The number of patient visits a week you need in order take home the minimum amount to survive _____

- The number of patient visits a week you'd like to see in order to live the life of your dreams _____

I urge you to do these estimations and calculations as best you can so that you can set clear and specific goals. And I urge you to write these goals down. People who write down their goals are 42% more likely to achieve them, according to a study conducted by Dr. Gail Matthews, a psychology professor at Dominican University of California. So, get specific with your goals, and then write them down! I think it harnesses and focuses your Qi in the direction of your dreams - a powerful thing.

I know, no one wants to talk finances, but here's the thing: it's an important piece to our life and our health. Our health? Yes. Our health. One of my friends and mentors, Dr. Emily Matuszewicz, teaches a class at Metropolitan State University of Denver called Holistic Health. In the curriculum she developed for this class, Dr. Emily spends several days discussing financial health.... in a Holistic Health class! I found that so surprising. "What do finances have to do with health?" I asked. What she said made so much sense: "What's a leading cause of illness? Stress. What's a leading cause of stress? Finances. Financial health, therefore, is directly related to our overall health and wellbeing." Boom - mind blown. That forever changed my perspective.

Being financially sound is good for your health and the health of your business.

The math and the money are what transform your dreams from vague figments of your imagination into a fully manifested plan. It's like magic, what can happen when you see the math written down on a page. It harnesses, focuses, and amplifies your Qi, your dreams, your vision, and your actions. I see its transformative power in the Start Your Acupuncture Clinic business class I teach all the time.

Office space

Besides education, rent is the biggest cost when it comes to your acupuncture business expenses, so it's wise to be conservative with it.

It makes it far easier to make it through the first 6 months when you're building your brand and reputation and network, and probably not as busy as you'd like to be. It takes time to get established, to get referral sources and a marketing funnel into place to attract a steady stream of patients into your clinic.

If you're strapped with the huge overhead costs of paying for three treatment rooms when you're hardly using one room to full capacity, for example, this creates a huge financial burden. This means less money to take home for yourself. Instead, start small and plan to expand into a bigger space when the time comes. Starting small does not mean playing small.

Personally, I invested in building walls to create two treatment rooms and a waiting room in my clinic when I first started. Then, I rented the second treatment room out to a massage therapist, cutting my monthly rent in half. After a year, I was ready to move into two treatment rooms, and I was so happy to be able to do that seamlessly.

Your office space doesn't need to be huge or fancy, so long as it's professional. Keep it clean without making it look cold and sterile. It can be cozy and it can be beautiful, but please make it professional. This will have a huge impact on your success.

I know it can feel annoying that our office space could have an effect on our success. It seems like our skills and the results of our treatments should be the sole determining factor on our success, doesn't it? Unfortunately, that's just not reality.

Of course, you do need to be a good practitioner and get good results in order to succeed, but that's not ALL you need. In reality, a number of other factors that have nothing to do with your results also affect your success. What factors? In a nutshell, all the factors that contribute to the general vibe around you that says, "I'm a professional, you're in good hands".

There are many elements that contribute to this feeling that you're a professional who can be trusted, and your office space is one of those elements. A big one. So, make sure that's what it communicates – that you're a professional. It can be small, but make sure it's not cluttered, and make sure it's well-organized and clean. Make it feel good. And don't just make it feel good to you and your personal aesthetic preferences, try to make it appeal to your potential patients as well.

How will they feel about tapestries hanging? Will they like it or will it make them think of Phish shows in college and perhaps hurt your perceived professionalism?

How will they feel about a big Buddha statue? Will it give them the (erroneous, but not uncommon) assumption that TCM is a religion and somehow in conflict with their own religious practices? Or will they find it soothing, like a spa atmosphere?

How will they feel about mag champa incense billowing from your space? Will it relax them? Or will it make them feel like they stumbled into a hippy head shop?

I recommend taking some time to think about the archetypal patient you'd most like to work with. What is that person like, what are they looking for, and what will make them feel comfortable?

There's no right answer to the above questions; it will depend on your target demographic, your location, and your space. I want you to just give it some thought. You're running a business. And it's about you, but it's not *only* about you - it's there to serve your patients.

Here are some things that are for sure *don't do's*: have dirty cups lying around and cluttering your waiting room or work space. Dusty surfaces. Stacks of paperwork on your reception desk. Stacks of dirty laundry. You get the idea. You're in healthcare, and being clean is crucial to making people feel safe.

Being professional

One common and easy-to-fix mistake I see acupuncturists making that dampens their growth is simply not being professional in their communications, marketing, and the systems they use to run their offices. No matter what kind of marketing you do, if you are not professional, you will undermine all of your efforts to build trust and credibility and attract and retain patients.

Acupuncture is hard to understand; it's scary because it involves needles. It's not part of the conventional medical system, so people can feel skeptical and uncertain about it. They are asking themselves, "Am I in the right place?" "Can this person really help me?" You want everything about their experience with you to be communicating a resounding "yes!" Yes, you are in good hands. Yes, we will take care of you. Studies and surveys show that it often takes eight to twelve treatments for patients to get results with acupuncture, so you can't simply rely on your great results to build trust and credibility because something has to make people want to stick around long enough to get results in the first place.

Imagine you're a potential client; there are two acupuncturists in your neighborhood, and you are deciding which one to see. One of them has a professional website with answers to your questions and well-lit and relevant photos, and they return your call or email promptly. The other one has a janky, confusing website with random photos of needles and sticks and twigs and people with red backs. When you left them a voicemail, it seemed to be their personal cell phone, and they didn't get back to you for days.

Clearly, you'd feel safer with the more professional one, right? I know, I know, it seems unfair because our website skills, design skills, and appearance have nothing to do with our diagnosis and herbal prescribing skills. You could be an amazing practitioner and have a janky website. You should be judged on your results, not all that other, less relevant stuff.

But here's the thing: People can't judge you on your results until they've committed to your care for many treatments. People don't know what needling should feel like. They don't know how spot-on your diagnosis is. They don't know how beautifully poetic your prescription and treatment plan is. They can't judge you on those things.

So, they're going to judge you based on the more visible and easy to assess things instead. To have a prospering practice requires that you are considered credible and relatable, and that you earn the trust of the people you'd like to serve - quickly.

Are you and your practice professional? Ask yourself this and be very honest. Being professional is hugely important if you want to grow a busy practice.

Being professional doesn't mean being stiff or stuffy. It doesn't mean you have to have anal retentive attention to detail or be super cautious and frugal. It just means having qualities, behaviors, and a way of conducting yourself and your business that create an optimal customer experience so that your patients want to do business with you again and tell everyone how wonderful you are. Being professional makes your life and your patients' lives a lot easier.

As healthcare practitioners, we have a unique hurdle to overcome. Health is different than other industries because it has a high trust requirement. People aren't just buying something from us, they are trusting us with their health! Building a high level of trust, authority, and connection and then inviting them to work with you, rather than trying to "sell" or pressure them with a discount is a far more effective way to attract patients.

If you market in the wrong way and inadvertently hurt rather than build trust, it can send the wrong message and have the opposite effect. It can make you seem desperate; it sends the message that you're not busy, and therefore not very good. You need to market and communicate in a way that sends the right message to people - that you are an expert they can trust, that you understand their problems, and that you are the solution that can help them. Simply being professional, in your marketing and in the way you run your practice, helps build trust and credibility, and that alone will make growing your clinic far easier. So, I hope I've really driven it home - you've got to be professional.

How to build your professionalism:

- You must have a professional and convenient location and a clean, attractive office space.

- You must dress appropriately and in clean clothes (as a rule of thumb, I recommend dressing to reflect the attire of the majority of your patients. Are they in business attire? Then I think you should reciprocate that. Are they casual? Then I think it'd be appropriate for you to be similarly casual).

- You must be well groomed. No perfume or cologne, as many of our patients are sensitive to smells. No body odor.

- You must be organized. Online scheduling is a godsend for your practice. It can act like a receptionist at a fraction of the price. It schedules people and sends reminder emails.

- Your intake paperwork is often your patients' first impression of your office. Make sure it's organized, concise, and not overwhelming. Use the same legible and professional font throughout all of your paperwork.

- You must use language and vocabulary that your patients understand.

- You must have a professional email address, preferably one that includes your domain name. katybaby@yahoo.com doesn't qualify. Neither does 1981KA@msn.com. If you don't have a website, then at least your name: Katiealtneu@gmail.com.

- You need a website that doesn't suck. If you don't have a website, get one! There are easy and super-affordable ways to do this yourself without hiring an expert: check out Squarespace, Weebly, Wix, and Wordpress, to name a few.

- Have professional photographs of yourself. A grainy photo of you in your pajamas with your dog is not going to inspire a lot of confidence.

- Obtain and showcase specific testimonials rather than general testimonials. "Katie was great. She really helped." isn't as impactful and specific as "Katie helped my back pain in 3 months. I tried everything before her, and nothing helped except her acupuncture!" This will carry a lot of weight, and it illustrates how you can help people.

First impressions

The old adage is true: You never get a second chance to make a first impression. What is the first thing you want your patients to experience? What's the first impression you want them to have? In what kind of mood should your introduction put them? These choices aren't driven only by what you say. Moods can be set by lighting, music, décor, clothing you're wearing, or the entrance you make. Within the first few seconds of meeting you, people will classify you somewhere in their minds and judge whether they will be able to connect with you or not. We humans are social animals and evolved to do this subconsciously and instantaneously.

Scan your office: Would decluttering and simplifying your space make it feel more peaceful or professional? Would adding some warmth with a plant or candle make it feel more approachable? Take some time to consider how it feels and the impression it makes. It doesn't need to be an expensive fix; I think that in general, less is more, and simplifying our space is the best way to go to make it feel more elevated.

Life isn't just "happening" to you. you're creating your world with every thought, every action, every word you speak.

Be aware that part of their first impression formed about you has already been made before they even enter your office. Consider all the communications you sent before the appointment. What was your website like? Your reminder email? Your paperwork? Your bio? Since all the interactions leading up to their visit create part of their first impression, make sure you've framed them appropriately. Here are some quick action steps to up your impression game:

- Revisit your bio on your website. Is it clear, concise, and also personal? Too often, we fill it with jargon and credentials that feel stuffy and impersonal, missing a crucial opportunity to connect with our potential patient who is curious to find out about us. Read it out loud and ask yourself – does it even sound like you? Rewrite it if necessary. Usually, just making the jargon and credentials more concisely written, adding in a first line and a last line that are more personal and welcoming are all that is needed, so it doesn't need to take long to do this.

- Look at your paperwork. Do all your forms use the exact same font? If not, choose a font that feels most like your branding on your logo or website or business card, and use that one consistently on all your forms. That's a quick and easy way to increase your perceived professionalism.

- Look at your reminder email (if you use a scheduling system that does this). Those systems often come with pre-formatted welcome emails, but usually, we can edit them. Does yours sound professional, concise, friendly, and like "you" (not too stuffy)? If not, then edit it so that it sounds like what you'd say when you are actually writing to a patient.

Those are some quick and easy ways to raise your perceived professionalism and increase the joy of working with you from the very beginning of a patient's journey in your care!

Standards of Service

These are the basic standards of service that are essential to establish your credibility.

- Quality of service and treatment
- Responsiveness. Your patients expect you to be responsive. They expect you to respond to their calls and emails in a timely manner.
- Client importance. It's essential to always make your patients feel important. You want to make them feel like the sun rises and shines just for them, because it does, if you want a prospering practice. You want everything about you and your clinic to say, "You're in the right place. You can trust us. We're pros. You're in good hands."

Which brings us perfectly to the next topic....

Chapter 8

Creating the Identity and Feel of your Clinic Brand

The name of your clinic and your logo are a big part of this (I dive into how to choose a name and logo for your clinic in my How To Start Your Acupuncture Clinic course), but I'm not going to cover choosing a name or logo here because many readers will already have this in place, and I want to stress all the other things that go into your brand that often get overlooked.

What is a brand? Your brand is everything that subconsciously signals and radiates the values you represent.

Having a cohesive brand instantly elevates the professionalism of your business and it's the easiest way to immediately indicate to strangers, "This is what I represent. This is who I am. You can trust me. This is what I'm about. I'm a pro."

It allows you to establish an emotional and almost instinctive connection with potential patients who come across your business. It allows you to attract the right type of patients for you, who you want to work with. And it allows you to express your unique vision, mission, style, flair, and passions.

"To be nobody but yourself - in a world which is doing its best, night and day, to make you everybody else - means to fight the hardest battle which any human being can fight"

— E.E. Cummings

Branding is done with your logo design, your colors and your fonts, and it's present in your logo, your website, your brochures, your business cards, everything. But it's also way MORE than just logo design, colors, and looking pretty.

Here's what I want to stress about branding. Your brand is really what you make people FEEL when they land on your website or your social media feed, walk into your clinic, or look at your intake paperwork or business card. Branding is what you're expressing and conveying to them; what you're making them FEEL, with not just your visuals, but with your VOICE as well – your tone, communication style and what you say. It's the personality of your brand and clinic.

So, give some thought to how you want to make people FEEL. If you already have a logo in place, look at it objectively and think, "How will this make my current and potential patients FEEL?"

I recommend working with a graphic designer because they are trained in how visuals (such as colors and fonts) make people feel. For example, an ephemeral cursive font expresses something different than a modern or bold font. Start looking around at other businesses' logos and fonts, and think to yourself, "How does this make me feel? What is this communicating?".

Some examples of things that might be communicated through a brand are, "we are joyful," "we are trustworthy," "we are modern," "we are classic and time-tested," "we are calm," "we are inspiring," and "we are natural." There is so much that you can communicate with images, fonts, colors, and the tone of your voice.

Think about how you want to make people feel, and think about WHO you want to resonate with. Design your branding for them, and not just what you want.

For example, if you want to work with older people, then you may keep in mind what will resonate with them (perhaps using larger fonts, for example). If you want to work with athletes, think about what would resonate with them (images of people doing athletic things, perhaps); and if you want to focus on fertility and women's health, think about what would resonate with them and instantly signal to them that you're the perfect fit (perhaps choosing softer colors, for example). Can you see how it might be different for each of these groups of people?

Design your brand so that you like it, but also make it so that the people that you most want to work with will also like it. And think about how you want to make them feel.

Look for inspiration - inspiration is everywhere. It's in nature, in photos of living rooms or bedrooms, photos of weddings, everywhere. Look for images of the feeling you want to conjure up with your clinic and branding. Find images that resonate with you, and ask yourself, "Why do I like this, and how is it making me feel?" That can be a big source of inspiration for you around which you can build your clinic branding.

you don't need to find
your voice. you have a voice.
you just need to stop
worrying about what other
people think when you use it.

Here are some questions to ask yourself:

- What's my mission/passion, and whom do I want to serve?
- What few words do I want associated with my clinic? (Maybe it's "natural," "health," "athlete," "ancient," "fertile," "trusted," "vibrant," "hope," "medical," "friendly," or "calm," for example.)
- Where do I want my brand vibe to fall between these characteristics:
  - Masculine/feminine
  - Simple/intricate
  - Grey/colorful
  - Conservative/extravagant
  - Approachable/authoritative
  - Necessity/luxury
  - Fun/serious
  - Professional/causal
  - Modern/classic
  - Sporty/elegant
  - Extreme/safe

Branding isn't just visual; it's also how you communicate your "voice" and your tone. It's embodied in the way you write on your website, social media, and brochures. Do you want to use an authoritative tone or a friendly, encouraging tone? What would fit your business, your personality, and your ideal patients better? Do you want a sophisticated and subtle tone, or a blunt, bold, no-

nonsense tone? Do you want to feel like someone's doctor or someone's BFF?

Here's another thing I want to stress about branding. It's wise to blend both being strategic and being yourself. What feels simultaneously like "you" and comes natural to you, and what feels like the vibe that would resonate with the patients you most want to work with, and the feelings you'd like to inspire in your patients and potential patients. Aim to strike a balance between being yourself and communicating mindfully to your potential patients. It will feel more in alignment with you, make marketing easier for you, and make you feel authentic.

I encourage you to let your personality come out a bit. Let people feel *you* in your branding. It will cultivate a much stronger connection between you and your current and potential patients. I made this common mistake when I first started out of not letting myself be "me". I tried really hard to sound professional, but I went about it in the wrong way. I used the royal "we" all over my website, even though it was just me back then. I sounded stuffy, almost like a computer or robot in my website copy instead of speaking/writing the way a real person talks – for example, I wouldn't use contractions ("is not" instead of "isn't"), which sounded robotic and fake.

In this day and age, being conversational with our writing (on our website and in our blog posts or social media posts) is much more compelling. It's easier to read, it's more inviting, and it develops connection way faster. Speak in plain conversational language. Relax your language. We need to be professional by using correct spelling and grammar, but we do NOT need to sound like robots. We should aim to sound like ourselves. And people will feel this from us and feel connected to us, and therefore trust us more easily.

Think about the tone that you want to relate to your patients with and what will resonate with the people you really want to work with. Let your personality shine through. In our type of work especially, which involves personal connections and close relationships, we don't need to invent or fabricate a brand personality. We just need to articulate and harness the best parts of our own true personality.

Your brand is your personality. Your personality is your brand. It's the only thing that you have a monopoly on. It's how you make yourself and your services unique from the acupuncturist down the street. When people want acupuncture from *you* because they know you, that's the ultimate edge. And to be clear, you don't have to act like you're better than other acupuncturists. The edge comes simply from having a connection - the know-like-trust factor.

You don't need to find or create your brand from thin air, just be yourself - but mindfully! Especially because our business is so personal, you are the face of your business. How great is that! It makes it feel so much easier, authentic, and rewarding. But many of us (including myself in the beginning) put up veils of what we think we "should" be, and hide behind a façade of professionalism by mimicking what everyone else is doing.

I'm sure people who meet you in real life like you and want to work with you. Are you embodying that same personality in your website and marketing? You can't meet one-on-one with every person, so you need to make your online presence work for you. That's what good, authentic, clear, and consistent branding does for you.

What stops you from putting yourself, your true personality, and your perspective on your website? I see this fear of visibility, of being seen, of allowing ourselves to take up space hold acupuncturists back (myself included). So, it's worth exploring. In case it's helpful to possibly stir up some of your own reflections, thoughts and experiences around this, I'll share some of my own fears that I've grappled with.

I was afraid of not being taken seriously. And I thought I had to speak and act in a polished and formal way in order to be taken seriously and seen as professional. I was afraid that people would think I was "woo-woo-ey," and that acupuncture was not legitimate, so I overcompensated with robotic, stuffy writing. But when is the last time you wanted to work with someone because they were stiff and formal? Never. I'd say conversational is the new professional. Once I realized that, and the fact that the world is just made of people that are dying to connect and relate, I was able to let my personality shine through more in my writing. Getting clarity around myself, my passion, my values, my strengths, and my perspective also helped me break my reliance on "shoulds" and vague, stuffy, professionalism. It helped me to step into my confidence.

I was also afraid of turning people off or alienating people who disagree or take offense to me and my opinions. I would never want to offend or alienate anyone, but I had to give that fear up. There is absolutely no brand or artist or food that is for everyone. Trying to be for everyone is a surefire way to blend in and be for no one - to resonate with no one. Connect with no one. I have to remind myself frequently that I'm coming from an intention of being of service and that my professional opinion and experience has the potential to really help someone, so I shouldn't hold back out of fear of turning someone off.

"She's unstoppable, not because she didn't have failures or doubts, but because she continued on despite them."

— Beau Taplin

I also, in my lack of confidence and clarity, mistakenly thought that there's only one way to have personality, like sass or arrogant confidence, for example, which are certainly not "me". Because I didn't have those personalities, I thought I suffered from "no personality syndrome". If you're like me, thinking that you're boring… ask yourself this: Do people in real life think you're boring? No. I bet they don't. So, share what makes you happy, mad, challenged, fired up. Share what you stand for; share your journey. Those things make you interesting and "unboring." And people will want to work with you because they feel connected to you. They will know you're not a robot, that you're not perfect, and that you're like them. AND you're an expert at what you do, and can help them!

We all have a collection of things and experiences that make us who we are. You've got to uncover and hone in on those. You could do an online personality test (like the Meyers Briggs test) or Google writing prompts. These may open up a floodgate and help you realize how many cool personality traits, quirks, stories, and lessons you have to share. And then purposefully let them shine in your branding.

I think the biggest obstacle, which was present for me as well, is the fear of being judged. I think this might be the biggest thing that holds us back. Check in, how present is this for you now? We all have this, accept it. We're social beings. Accept and acknowledge it. We all do. It doesn't make you less than. And what you resist persists.

Instead, step into being of service, even to one person. People will be forced to judge you for being of service, helping others, and doing what you love. How can someone think negatively of you for that?

Don't make it about you. It's about serving; contributing. The secret to living is giving. If you have something bigger than your fear that you're working for, it's far easier. Hone in on what you care about more than your fear of being judged or your fear of failure. I believe motive does matter. And courage is a muscle... practice it, grow it. It gets easier.

Most of us become acupuncturists because we wanted meaning, connection, and the chance to touch lives. We're amazing at this inside the treatment room. Why don't we bring those things into our marketing too? How do we do that? As Brené Brown teaches, we accomplish that by being vulnerable. By allowing ourselves to be seen. Brené Brown is a researcher on shame at the University of Houston and the author of several books including *Daring Greatly* and *The Gifts of Imperfection*. Based on years of research and interviews, she found that "Vulnerability is the birthplace of love, belonging, joy, courage, empathy, and creativity. It is the source of hope, empathy, accountability, and authenticity. If we want greater clarity in our purpose or deeper and more meaningful spiritual lives, vulnerability is the path."

It's all about connection. If you were looking at two perfectly similar offers, you would choose to buy or work with the one that you felt the most connected to, right? We want to work with and purchase from the businesses that we feel the most connected to. How can we both create more connection AND scale to reach more people? How can you show people who you haven't yet met that you're willing to connect one on one? That you're willing to show up? That you care?

By actually being yourself throughout all of your branding. You are your biggest selling point. People want to connect with the heart behind the work. A *business* sells and markets a service or product - a service or product that is a just like all the similar services or products around. That's not really what I want to be, do you? On the other hand, a *brand* is a personality that shifts hopes and dreams. It's what people connect to, fall in love with, and get excited about. Businesses are constantly marketing and selling. Brands don't have to do that.

If you've connected with people, they will be dying to work deeper with you. You don't need to speak to everyone, just your ideal patients that you really want to work with. So, they see/hear your message and think, "'Without a doubt, I know this person is for me."

Branding is a sacred opportunity to really be ourselves, and to do it mindfully and on purpose. When we can fully articulate who we are, who we serve, how and why we help them, and what we can help them accomplish, we'll find abundance and fulfillment of our own. That's how we can be of the most service to the world. When we take full responsibility for how we're showing up in the world – really really show up, Brené Brown style – we create the perfect level of vulnerability needed to forge meaningful connections with patients . That's what I LOVE helping acupuncturists do in my Attract More Acupuncture Patients course, and it's why marketing can feel surprisingly spiritually fulfilling.

Be yourself, connect, be different, have a point of view, hit a nerve, inspire, connect. Make sure your brand and your tone are in alignment with who you are AND will resonate with your ideal patients. It's helpful to write down the qualities and feelings you're aiming inspire to encompass your brand.

And then be consistent. Consistency is key – use that voice on all of your materials: your website, social media, intake forms, business cards, etc. It hurts trust if you lack consistency, or if your brand and voice feel different from what it actually feels like to come into your clinic and receive treatment from you. It needs to all feel aligned, authentic, and consistent. This builds trust, confidence, connection, and loyalty.

How do you want to show up for people? How can you show up *truly* as yourself, and most helpfully for the people whom you want to serve?

Here are some action steps that may help you:

- Ask five of your closest friends and family to describe your personality. It doesn't have to be a big, time-consuming analysis - a simple list of a handful of words that describe you is fine.

- Make a list of qualities, values, or feelings that you'd like your brand to radiate – that you'd like to inspire in your current and potential patients.

- Find the overlap so that it feels like "you," and it conveys what you'd like to convey. Make a simple list of your brand "voice" or "vibe" or "qualities".

- Read your website, your latest social media posts, blog posts or marketing materials. Does it sound like you and the brand "voice" you're going for? Can you make some tweaks on your website so that this comes out a little more authentically? Moving forward with social media posts, blog posts, or marketing materials, keep this "voice" in mind. Keep that list you made handy and revisit it as you create new posts or marketing materials.

The key to getting
more patients is
to "get" your patients.

Chapter 9

Your Best Communication Strategy

If you believe in what you do and you know that your services help people improve their lives, then you have an *obligation* to make sure that you attract the people who need you the most.

Marketing, which is too often the weakest area of business for acupuncturists, is the area of your business that has the most dramatic impact and potential leverage for your growth, success, and impact on others' lives. Marketing doesn't have to be your greatest passion. Hopefully, acupuncture and TCM are what inspire you the most. But, in order to touch lives, you've got to embrace this.

A lot of acupuncturists think that if they just get amazing results, patients will be lining up and knocking down their door. They think they can rely only on results and word-of-mouth referrals as a consequence of those results. So, they spend hundreds and even thousands of dollars to take a new seminar or learn a new technique, hoping that maybe they will get busy. But typically this is not the thing that will get you busy.

People don't buy because
what you do is awesome.
People buy because it
makes them feel awesome.

Studying is great, continuing to learn is great, and you do need to be an excellent practitioner, but it isn't going to be the thing that will actually grow your business. You could be the best in town, using amazing needle technique, crafting beautiful herbal formulas, achieving dramatic results in your patients, and STILL not be attracting the number of patients you want! And that sucks!

But if you think about it, it makes sense – if you can't figure out how to effectively attract people to your business and elegantly turn them into retained patients, you're finished. It doesn't matter how great of an acupuncturist or herbalist you are if no one knows about you, trusts you, or gets you.

So, here's the insight I really want to share with you. If you have a product or service that makes the world a better place (which you do), then it is your moral responsibility to get your business in front of as many people as possible.

And right now, there are thousands of people with problems that you have solutions for. You have what they need! They just don't know it yet! So, here's the thing: It's not their job to find you, it's your job to reach them!

For many acupuncturists, the word "marketing" conjures up images of slick advertisements, pushy salespeople and big budgets poured into highly visible campaigns. But that's not the kind of marketing I'm talking about. Our marketing can and should be authentic and feel good.

As healthcare practitioners, we have a unique hurdle to overcome. Health is different than other industries because it has a high trust requirement. People aren't just buying a widget or a shoe from us, they are entrusting us with their health! They are entrusting us with needles, and taking a leap on a form of care that is outside of conventional medicine.

If you market in the wrong way, it can send the wrong message and have the opposite of the desired effect. For example, if you just discount your services, this can seem desperate, sending the message that you're not busy, and therefore not very good. Potential patients are likely to think that if you're discounting your services, then you must not be very busy. In turn, if they think you're not busy, then you must not be very good. I know that's not true – there are so many gifted acupuncturists who aren't busy – but it's an association and assumption people make.

Good marketing focuses on communicating the right message to people - that you are an expert they can trust, that you understand their problems, that they don't have to keep living the way they are living, that there is a solution, and that you are the solution that can help them.

Good marketing is about: 1) deeply knowing who you are and what you have to offer and 2) speaking to the deep desires of the specific group of people who will appreciate it most. The goal is to communicate to them in a way that makes them *inspired and eager to take action*. It should make them eager to refer their friends; eager to come back and keep coming back.

Effective marketing is about resonating with people. It's about creating genuine connection. Genuine connections create change in people's hearts and minds. Marketing, whether you realize it or not, is trying to persuade people to change. You're moving people to go from uninformed to informed, from uninterested to interested, and from being stuck to being unstuck. You are also asking people to do something with the information you're conveying, which makes marketing persuasive.

Resonance causes change, not coercion or slimy, slick sales people. Resonating with people so that they see your message and think, "Yes, I instinctively know that that is true and that it's for me" creates change. That's good marketing.

But here's the kicker: People don't need to tune themselves to you – you need to tune your message to them. Skilled marketing requires you to understand their hearts and minds, and to create a message that resonates with what's in their hearts from a place of alignment, confidence and authenticity. They will be moved if you send them a message that is tuned to their needs and desires. Your job is to make your potential patients "get" you and what you offer. But in order to do that, you have to "get" them - their problems, their needs, and their desires.

I'm going to help you figure out how to communicate what you do in a way that really connects and resonates with patients.

I want to introduce you to a few concepts that we'll talk about in more depth.

Virtually all marketing activities can be divided into 3 categories:

1. Your market – I think of your market as your people. Your WHO. Your market is made up of people who are not only the *most likely to buy, want and benefit from* your services, but also the people you would most love to work with. The people you want to serve. Most practitioners make the mistake of offering their services to the general population without first determining who their niche market is (you'll learn how to do this in the next section). Once you've identified your market, you'll research further to understand their wants and desires.

2. Your message – your message is what you are telling people you can do for them. It should speak directly to your market's wants and desires.

One of the biggest mistakes I see acupuncturists make with marketing is that they are too focused on themselves. The truth is, successful marketing is client-focused, meaning it is *all about your patients*. While you should be yourself and harness your own personality and perspective, the focus of your marketing content should be on your patients.

Your communications should be focused on your patient's goals, dreams or objectives, showing them how you can help them get from where they are to where they want to be (or where they think they want to be initially) better than any of the other options out there.

Dale Carnegie once said that, "When dealing with people, remember you're not dealing with creatures of logic, but with creatures of emotion, creatures bristling with prejudice and motivated by pride and vanity." Carnegie's statement contains an important truth that is all too often overlooked by practitioners. When it comes down to it, most people's buying decisions are selfish!

People want to know, "What's in this for me?" "Where's the value?" "Is this worth it?" "Why should I spend my time, energy and money on this?" A compelling message that motivates your market to pay attention and take action must take this "selfishness" into account.

What message have you been telling people? Is it all about *them* and what *they* want and care about, or is it all about *you*? Here are four questions to ask yourself regarding your current message on your website and marketing materials:

A. Does it help people clearly and specifically see the value of what I can do for them?

B. Does it show them how I can help them feel better in an area of their life where they're experiencing pain and desire a solution?

C. Does it show them very explicitly why I'm the best choice for them?

D. Does it answer these questions:

    a. Why should I buy this?

    b. Why should I buy it from you?

Whoever answers these questions clearly and authentically will have a full and thriving practice.

3. Your medium – your medium is your delivery mechanism. This is how you get your message in front of your market.

Your medium could be social media, your website, email, direct mailing, radio, flyers, classes, other health providers, conversations in the treatment room, etc. The more capable it is of connecting to and resonating with your target market, and the more aligned it is with you and your brand, the better your chances of success.

Imagine there are two acupuncturists. One of them – in person and on his website – communicates that he is a licensed acupuncturist, he's been in practice 9 years, he has three treatment rooms, he treats all kinds of things and that anyone and everyone can benefit from acupuncture. He's actually great at treating IBS, back pain, and anxiety, but he doesn't say that specifically because he doesn't want to turn someone off who has something other than those ailments. He tries marketing messages (on Facebook ads or flyers) that say "Feel better now. 25% off your first acupuncture visit". But they don't get much traction, and he feels like advertising doesn't work.

The other acupuncturist – in person and on her website – communicates that she loves treating IBS and digestive complaints. She explains that there are so many natural solutions to these problems, even when western medicine doesn't have answers and nothing is officially "wrong" or diagnosed, and she loves helping patients with these. She has blog posts explaining her process that give specific diet and lifestyle tips. She has specific testimonials showing success stories overcoming IBS. And even though she can also treat all kinds of other things from anxiety to back pain, when she does a Facebook ad or flyer, she chooses specific message that says, "finally overcome IBS, even if you feel like you've already tried everything, so that you can hike all day without worrying about where the closest bathroom is."

Who do you think gets more traction and attracts more patients? The acupuncturist who is vague and general? Or the acupuncturist who clearly and consistently conveys the benefits of her care? Whose message strongly resonates with this subset of people? Her message resonates with people. It's clear and compelling, and it inspires people to action.

The trick to figuring out your best message is to get specific.

Figuring out a resonant message takes some thought. In order to resonate with people and clearly convey how you can help them, you've got to get specific. You must show them how their life will be improved by what you do in a way that they'll understand and care about enough to actually want to take action!

The average person doesn't understand what you mean by "balance" or "boost qi". The average person also doesn't realize how connected stress is to their specific health concern. In order for the average person to understand the value of your care for them, they need you to specifically lay it out.

In order to do that, you've got to narrow the "market" that you're focusing on communicating with. You've got to back it up a bit. Acupuncture can help pretty much ANYONE with anything and EVERYTHING, right? That's what I think, at least. But to say that in your marketing wouldn't be even remotely effective. A horribly ineffective marketing message would be something along the lines of, "We can help almost anyone with anything!" That falls so flat. It gets no one's attention. It resonates with no one (aside from we acupuncturists who would cheer it on like "darn right it can!") But to our potential patients, it means nothing, it seems hokey, and it's drowned out by the noise of life.

A more compelling marketing message is one that catches someone's attention because it speaks to their needs and helps them self-identify that it is decidedly meant for them, resonates with their needs, clearly shows them a path, lets them know there's hope, and inspires them to action. An example of a good marketing message would be something like, "Natural treatments for IBS" or "Effective, natural treatments for all types of infertility". These work because they are clear, they use the exact word that people with that condition relate to (rather than "digestive problems" in the place of IBS, for example), and they instill hope, which is exactly the resonance that's needed to inspire them to action.

Let's turn the table around and put yourself in the "layman's" shoes. Let's say we're talking about a therapy that we don't really know much about - let's use "hydrotherapy" as an example. Sounds like it involves water, but I'm not quite sure exactly what's involved or what it can treat. And let's also say that I suffer from arthritis. If I see an ad or website saying "Hydrotherapy – helping you feel your best," it won't really get my attention or compel me to take action, because it's not clear that it can actually help me specifically with what I'm dealing with. Now imagine I saw an ad or website that said, "Effective natural relief for arthritis – hydrotherapy!" Now *that* would get my attention. We need to get specific, paint a picture people can personally relate to, and even use the exact language that they use to self-identify with a problem. That's how we expand the circle of awareness of how acupuncture can benefit people.

So, in order to have a compelling message, we need to understand why people would want to get acupuncture.

> Why do people choose to get acupuncture? What are the benefits for them? What are some specific ways you help improve peoples' lives? What is an outcome of working with you?

Now I know that this is a HUGE question, because I think acupuncture can help almost anyone and any problem.

So, in order to make this exercise easier and more useful, we need to back up a bit.

Let's not ask those questions about EVERYONE who could benefit from acupuncture. That would be so huge and hard to define!! Let's think about it in terms of YOUR ideal patients and target market. Why would THEY come to you for your services? What are the benefits they will receive?

In order to do this effectively, we will need to identify your target market and ideal patient.

Why you need to identify your ideal patient(s) and target market(s).

Get particular about who you want to work with. Don't be so general or generic and take on trying to attract everyone, though you may be tempted to market to everyone with the assumption that the more people you market to, the more patients you'll get.

When I first started out, I was so enthusiastic about helping people that I wanted to help everyone with all ailments. I knew there were so many people who need and can benefit from acupuncture, and thought crowds of people would be banging down my door. But it turns out, patients didn't fall from the sky. I was baffled and frustrated because I knew I could help so many people. I really thought it would be easy. But that didn't happen.

I didn't have a clearly defined target market or ideal patient so I couldn't make an effective marketing message. I was staying too general. It diluted my message, so my marketing didn't resonate with anyone.

While *narrowing* your market to gain *more* patients may seem counterintuitive, that's exactly what you need to do to successfully get more patients. You may feel like you are limiting yourself, but you will end up expanding your market because more people will flock to you.

It's tricky to appeal to the broader market while deeply connecting and resonating with everyone. It is a simple fact that the more you know about someone, the easier it is to communicate with them in the language that they understand and relate to. Once you know your people, your target market or ideal patient, you will begin writing, marketing and communicating in a way that they feel heard and understood. They will trust you as an expert who can help them. When you have made the effort to speak and write directly to your ideal patient, they will feel it. They will feel as though you truly know and understand their needs and desires – because you will.

All of this ties back to defining your ideal clients. Who are they? What is their pain point, what are you helping them with, and how are you clearly conveying to them that you are the answer to their problem? Determine which group of people is most likely to resonate with you, to need your services, and who you would love to work with – the group with which you can make the greatest impact.

Here's what I find so many acupuncturists doing to themselves. They feel like if they make their message specific, and believe me, I used to think this too, they will create a situation where someone who might have been interested in your services wouldn't come to them.

But when you make your message specific, you attract the people who you love to work with, who you want to support, and who you have the expertise and knowledge to help. You attract them easily, with less effort and expense. The big misconception is that if you remain general, then you will attract EVERYONE. Well, how's it working out for you?

When you generalize, you're not speaking to anyone specifically. It's not speaking to everyone like you think it is, it's actually speaking to no one. No one's connecting with you because you aren't speaking their language, you're not talking about their specific problems, and you're not hitting on their pain points. That's why you've got to decide – who do you want to serve? Who do you want to attract? Who is your ideal patient?

So, I want to ask you: Have you found yourself struggling with this? Have you found yourself not wanting to give clarity to your ideal patient or your marketing message because you're afraid of potentially not getting chosen by someone that otherwise would possibly choose you?

I want you to know that that's normal. And it's ok - it is hard. I also want you to know that you don't need to pick *one* specialty. You can pick several areas of focus. You can have several target markets and focuses. But every time you do a piece of marketing, you've got to get laser focused and specific on resonating with that ONE group. Otherwise it will fall flat.

Let's help you hone in on YOUR target market(s)

For each one of us acupuncturists, the answer to this question is different because we bring our own unique background. We may have the same degree and certification, but our history and life experiences are what make us unique. And we need to bring that into our marketing.

Don't just choose a target market based on what you think you *should* choose, choose one that interests and excites you. Otherwise, you'll end up bored and frustrated in your practice, and your marketing will fall flat. When you choose a target market you're passionate about, your practice will feel good and easy, and it will bring you joy. And marketing it will too.

when you're speaking
to everyone, you're
speaking to no one

A common mistake acupuncturists make is to THINK they've identified an ideal patient when in reality they haven't. So often I ask my acupuncture students to identify their ideal patient. A common response is something along the lines of, "My ideal client is someone who wants more energy to do things in life that they love. I'm going to help them boost their energy."

That's an honorable goal, but it's still really generic because it doesn't ask these important questions: Who are you speaking to? Who are you going to be giving that energy to? Because who wants more energy? That really describes most of the population, doesn't it? I don't know about you guys, but when I fall into bed at night, I feel like I had a busy and full day, running my practice, serving my patients and chasing after my toddler. So, energy for me would mean something very specific, about a mom/business owner lifestyle. But if we dig a little deeper on this energy topic, to give you solid examples, we could talk about the specific types of people who need more energy.

Consider a corporate executive who works 80 hours per week. Now, this person may say, "I want more energy, I'm exhausted." Another example is a stay at home mom who has 3 kids under the age of 5, which makes me feel exhausted just thinking about. Or, it could be a woman going through menopause and experiencing hormone levels that are all over the place. Each and every one of these people need and want more energy. But the way you would speak to them, market to them, write your website, brochures, flyers, blog posts, and social media posts would all be very different. You would use different phrases and terminology for a stay-at-home mom than you would for a corporate executive who is working 80 hours a week.

New mantra: I am capable
of deeply understanding
my patients and potential
patients. When I can harness
that power and express
it in my marketing,
everything gets easier.

You could take that same solution, to increase energy levels, and based on how you speak about it, you could attract one of these individuals. But not all them. Because if you just said, "I can show you how to get more energy," none of these people are going to pay attention to you. It doesn't speak to them. They are exhausted. They want a quick fix. They want to know you have the answer, and that you can relate to them. They want to know you understand the world they are living in, and they want to know that you GET IT. It's a big difference depending on who you are speaking to.

Can you see how this changes your marketing message? Are you thinking about how your use of language and images can help or harm your message in certain scenarios? Can you see how you should be more specific, and how this makes a huge difference with your marketing?

You can still treat all of those different people; you don't have to turn people away. However, your marketing should speak to specific people in order to attract them while maintaining effectiveness.

Clarity breeds confidence. As you get more and more clear about who your target market is and you start speaking their language and developing your expertise just for them, your website and other marketing materials will confidently reflect this level of insight as well. And that all starts with your ideal client and your messaging.

What's the difference between a clear approach and a general one? With a clear approach, your social media posts, emails, website, and ads will be much more targeted. For example, let's say you were targeting IBS. Instead of being vague and general, you'd share social media posts about IBS and bloating, you'd have a specific page all about IBS on your website, you'd have blog posts about IBS, constipation, bloating, loose stools and so on, and your ads or talks would be targeted to IBS as well. This is huge. This is how you start getting the attention and interest of people who didn't even know they were in need of an acupuncturist. By getting specific and targeted and going deep instead of wide.

There are tons of people who need your services. And with customization and just a little clarity on whom you want to serve, you can attract way more patients. You want to learn everything about your ideal patient so that you can speak directly to their pain points - the things that keep them up at night - making sure to let them know how your solution and services answer their needs. That's how you'll get a ton of patients who want to work with you.

You can take this as far as you want to take it, meaning you don't need to apply this to more than you're comfortable with. Even applying it a little bit more than you currently do will benefit your marketing efforts. You don't need to rename your clinic. You don't even have to redesign your website if you don't want to, so don't let that fear or misconception stop you from moving forward with this. What you MUST do, at the very least, is use this to make your marketing efforts, ads, promotions, events, blog posts, and headlines more effective, actually WORKING to attract people. If you don't make sure that those are talking to specific pain points and resonating with your target market, then you're wasting your time and energy.

Let's help you identify and hone in on your ideal patient and target market. An easy place to start is with your current patients. You may find that most of your patients share common elements; it may be that these elements are naturally drawn to you. Perhaps your target market has already chosen you, and you just haven't realized it!

Below is a worksheet to walk you through the process of identifying your ideal patient.

List the possibilities that appeal to you, sit with them for a bit and then choose those that are calling most to you. Tune into your intuition, turn off your censor, and allow yourself to play and be curious. Remember, you're not limiting yourself here. You're not going to NOT serve people who don't fit into this neat little picture of your ideal patient. But identifying your target patient is going to allow you to create and implement far more effective marketing strategies. It will allow you to produce messages that resonate and speak to your audience on a deeper level.

Exercise 1: Consider your life experience and interests. What life situations or health challenges have you personally experienced or witnessed, and what situations do you identify with? Maybe you or a loved one suffered from a certain illness or health issue. *Maybe you're an avid runner or yogi, for example.*

_____

_____

_____

_____

Exercise 2: Think of all the different types of people or conditions who can benefit from acupuncture. Which of these groups do you most relate to or feel the most excitement about or passion for helping? Which group(s) are already part of your community?

Which areas would you be excited to learn more about? Which group(s) do you have the most knowledge about or experience in? Which groups do you get results with? *For example, maybe you're excited about working with running injuries and sports recovery.*

_____

_____

_____

_____

Exercise 3: You might as well be serving people who light you up. Look at your current patient base and ask yourself: Who do I look forward to seeing, and who do I enjoy being around? Who are the patients that don't feel like work to me? What patients have felt easy, fulfilling, AND fun for me? Look for trends in your patient base - what did they originally come in for? Write down some of the names that come to mind and their chief complaint, secondary complaint, qualities, or characteristics.

For example, maybe it's specifically women runners, and even more specifically, working moms who are also runners that seem to light you up the most.

_____

_____

_____

_____

Exercise 4: Look through the above 3 exercises and bring it all together. What showed up the most repetitively or strongly for you in the answers above? This, or these if there's more than one, are your target market(s):

_____

_____

_____

_____

Exercise 5: Instead of thinking about your market of potential patients as a group, imagine them each as individuals. This will help you to cultivate more empathy in your marketing message, because you will feel like it's directed at ONE person. WHO is one of your target patients? Describe what he or she is like. Get really creative with this one. List as many specific details as you can.

> *Example: "Jane Doe, a 44-year-old professional. She has two children and a dog. She's a runner, and her knees and ankles get achy. She also has difficulty falling asleep, and struggles with anxiety. She's health conscious, outdoorsy, smart, and driven. She does yoga once a week, runs around the park a couple times a week with her dog, goes for longer runs on the weekend, and is training for a half marathon. She knows she needs to embrace more self-care, but also feels like she doesn't have a ton of time for it. She works from home and makes $70,000 a year."*

There's no right or wrong answer. This is simply an exercise of empathy and imagination. You're trying to connect more deeply in order to resonate with one of the many people you could help.

Your turn. Describe whom you'd like to attract to your practice.

_____

_____

_____

_____

Identify the needs and desires of your target patient

Now that you've identified your target patient, let's dig a little deeper. You've got to understand what your ideal patients are looking for - what their problems and goals are.

Humans are more complex than just the broad strokes that define demographics: age, where they work, their geographic location, income level, or even chief complaint. In order to connect personally, you have to bond with what makes people human. Having my specific description of "Jane Doe" allows me to exercise my empathy and put myself in her shoes. It allows me to think more deeply about what her struggles and desires are, what would resonate with her, and how I could best serve her. That's why it's just an exercise. There's no right answer – it's just a process that helps you develop your empathy and creativity when trying to think deeply about your potential patients' needs.

If you want to fill your practice, you need to find out what your target market is really looking for. What's the biggest challenge, problem or concern for potential patients in your target market? What do they want for themselves in the future? What is important to them? What is it that they'd really like to avoid? What are they looking for?

The more connected you
are with your audience,
the more you'll be able
to resonate with them

In general, people want to be happy, healthy, and wealthy, and they want to look and feel good. No matter how spiritually enlightened people are, they primarily make purchases for those reasons. Can you get more specific, though? Do they want to run their half marathon pain-free? Do they want to sleep through the night so they feel more rested? Do they want to sleep through the night so they can heal and prevent injury? Do they want to sleep through the night so they can be more present and joyful with their family? Do they want to have a baby? Do they want to feel more in control of their health? Do they want to feel less anxious? Do they want to prevent their next migraine? Do they want to feel less bloated so they can feel confident and go on dates? Do they want to feel less bloated because it's difficult to focus on work when you're all bloated and distended? And so on.

You've got to understand what your ideal patients are looking for - what keeps them up at night. It's very important to get clear on this, because if you don't know what your potential patients are looking for, you won't know what to tell them about how you can help. You won't be able to inspire the hope they so need from you.

For example, your best marketing is *not* going to be a flyer that says "Try acupuncture!" or "Acupuncture works!" or even "Reduce stress" or "Relieve back pain!". For your target patient, marketing that catches their eye speaks to them on a deeper level. It might be something like, "Because mommies need nap time too" or "Because even runners need to rest" or "I want you to know there are natural solutions to IBS. You don't have to be bloated forever." Something that will make them think – oh my gosh, she gets me! And – oh my gosh, there's hope!

"A leader is a deal in hope"

— Napolean Bonaparte.

So is an acupuncturist.

We usually make offers that WE THINK are relevant. It's time to utilize your amazing ability to empathize, put your target market first and work to truly understand what *they know* is relevant to them. Then you can decide on what you're going to communicate to them that will most resonate with, interest, and inspire them. Your objective is to find the most relevant way to link your services to your market's top values and concerns.

Exercise 1: Keeping in mind the identity you created in the previous exercise to think empathetically about one of your target patients, what is your target patient looking for? *Example: In my case, they are looking for ways to support their body during training for a half-marathon.*

_____

_____

_____

Exercise 2: What are five of your target patient's urgent needs? What keeps them up at night? What problems must they solve right away? Example: Do they have knee pain and want to prevent injury? Do they need an alternative to their medications? Do they want to enhance their performance? Do they want to support their recovery so they can train harder?

_____

_____

_____

Exercise 3: What are five of your target patient's *deeper desires*? What would they like to move toward? What is lacking in their lives?

What's important to them? *Example: Do they want to win the race? Do they need a break from their busy schedule to nurture and care for themselves? Do they need to get a good night's sleep? Do they need to feel less overwhelmed, more clarity, joy, and focus? Do they need pain relief?*

_____

_____

_____

Here's a big hint: Do you know what generally *doesn't* keep people up at night? What is *not* an urgent need or deep desire? They are the exact things I used to say in my marketing (forehead smack). Things like "get to the root of your health problems", "healing, powered by you", "get back to yourself again", "align your health with nature", and vague things like that. I literally try to imagine someone lying in bed at night, worrying, and I ask myself, is this something someone would actually say to themselves?

Uncover the deeper benefits of your services

Once you really understand what your patients want and need, you can better **communicate the value** of what you can do for them and inspire them to take action. You can show them how their lives will be improved by what you do in a way that they'll understand and care about enough to actually want to take action.

You could provide the world's most life-changing services, but that won't guarantee your success in practice. *You've got to be able to communicate that value to your patients.*

It's easy to assume that we know what people want. Everyone would want to circulate blocked qi and restore balance to the body if they knew what that really meant for them. But that's a foreign language to most people! It's your job to translate that language into something meaningful and compelling that your patients can understand.

Remember: People, whether they're conscious of it or not, don't initially come to you for your services. They come to you for the results.

For example:

Don't sell me a restaurant dinner, sell me:

- an escape from the evening dishes
- a moment of romantic intimacy
- a great taste experience without any guilt

Don't sell me dance lessons, sell me:

- increased confidence for my child
- a feeling of belonging for my child as a part of a dance group
- an opportunity to learn discipline

Don't sell me acupuncture, sell me:

- the baby I've been longing for
- a sound night's sleep
- a faster recovery from surgery
- less bloating and more food freedom, without drugs
- and so on

"Hope is a good thing.
Maybe the best of things.
And no good thing ever dies."

— The Shawshank Redemption

What your patients really want is to experience the results of what you do. In other words, they want what your services will get them. So, think about your ideal patients, put yourself in their shoes, and ask the question, "What's in it for me?"

Before you can articulate this, however, you've got to first figure out what you're really offering your patients. You're not just offering acupuncture, you're offering so much more than that!!

Until you've clearly defined for yourself what you're REALLY offering and what the benefit behind the benefit is in concrete terms (especially when your services are unfamiliar or unorthodox to people), you won't be able to successfully market your services.

There are tons of ways to do this. Many acupuncturists sell the features of their services – the science of acupuncture, how it works, how it balances the hormone levels and relieves pain, how long they've been in practice, who they've trained with, what advanced seminars they've taken, etc., but they fail to highlight how it's going to benefit the patient. You need to articulate this result or benefit from either a physical, emotional, spiritual or financial perspective.

Will your potential patients be more willing to invest in your services if they believe that doing so would substantially increase the chances of conceiving? Of course they would. If that's your target patient's pain or problem, then you must communicate that you have the best solution for them.

To make it obvious for your potential patients, you need to uncover and demonstrate the benefits of working with you. Acupuncture is *technically* what your patients buy, but not what they *actually* buy.

They are buying tangible and intangible results – your patients are buying the effects your services have on their quality of life. This is what makes acupuncture worth the investment. For example, people are buying these results from you: peace of mind; feeling rested; being free from pain; being able to play with their kids; being able to focus at work; having a baby; winning the race; feeling beautiful; having a more active lifestyle.

Do you see how identifying the deeper benefits of your services allows you to speak to and touch people on a much deeper and more emotional level? People pay for a service to get the deeper benefits found in the results, not for the service itself. So, think about a few of the various problems you help people solve, and the deeper benefits that provides.

I also believe that the better acupuncturists get at communicating the value of what we do, the more effective we'll be at holding our own against the encroaching field of dry needling by physical therapists. Yes, perhaps it's important to educate people that we are also an energy medicine; perhaps it's important to educate people that dry needling is one of the forms of needling that some acupuncturists are trained in and that for many acupuncturists' styles, dry needling is the same thing. However, I believe that it would be most effective to say confidently and compassionately, "This is what we help."

The first question any new patient wants answered is, "How can you help me?".

Nope, it's not "What are your credentials and who are you?" – that comes second. They only care about that once they know you can help them. If you can't, frankly, they don't care about wasting their time learning about your credentials. And it's also not, "How does acupuncture work?".

In my early days in practice, I got hung up on the "how it works" question. Somehow, a simple question such as, "*How does acupuncture work?*" can make our brains short circuit, conjuring run-on sentences and making us sound like blundering idiots who don't understand our own medicine or how the body works. Not because we don't understand our own medicine or how the body works, but because it's so complex, and we know so much, and it can be difficult to condense all this knowledge down in a simple, concise, and clear manner.

You DO need to be able to answer that question in an intelligent and concise manner, and with vocabulary that the average person understands. I made an infographic about how to answer this, which can be found here: https://acuprosper.com/how-should-i-say-that/ In a nutshell, my preferred answer (although I tend to tailor it depending on who I'm talking to) is: "Acupuncture has been shown to increase circulation, decrease inflammation, relieve pain and muscle spasms, and increase T-cell count to stimulate the immune system. This is why acupuncture works well for so many things, from pain to anxiety and fertility." I like this because it doesn't include the word "Qi," which the layperson doesn't understand. Nor does it include the word "energy," which many people misunderstand. It's easy for the average Western mind to grasp, and I can back it all up with research.

The most crucial element is for each acupuncturist to be able to clearly communicate the value of their work - the answer to *why* people should care in the first place.

I've never even once had a patient sit in my intake chair after the initial intake and questioning process and refuse to get on the table without being told how it works first. People ask that question, but they ask it once they're on the treatment table, conversationally and out of curiosity – not as a barrier to receiving treatment. If I've fully communicated that I understand their problem and I feel somewhat confident and hopeful that I can help, then they are 100% game for treatment.

It's all about effectively communicating your value.

How to communicate your "Value"

If your marketing efforts aren't working at attracting people and converting them into patients, if your potential patients hesitate based on the cost of acupuncture, or if your patients aren't sticking around because of the cost, then this means you are not effectively communicating your benefits, which translates to VALUE for the patient.

Here's a marketer's definition of value:

$$VALUE = DESIRABILITY \ Divided \ By \ PRICE$$

In other words, the lower the price, the better VALUE it appears to have, which is common knowledge. But this is also true: the higher the desirability, the better value it appears to have.

The interesting thing about VALUE is that it's very subjective. I'll give you an example of just how subjective value is:

Beauty Counter is a natural body care line that has a much higher price point than other makeup brands. But they also have a huge, devoted, and growing following because they are actively educating people about the dangerous ingredients in most conventional beauty care lines. Once you understand how phthalates and parabens can disrupt our hormones and our health, suddenly, an all-natural phthalate- and paraben-free makeup line seems much more compelling and valuable, right? Suddenly, you're no longer looking at the cost of face cream; you're marveling at the benefits of those items.

Although the price stays the same, the perceived value goes up dramatically, following the formula VALUE = DESIRABILITY divided by PRICE.

To get more patients in the door, you don't need to lower your price to convey your value - you need to make sure your services appear highly desirable. You increase desirability by communicating the benefits and solutions you offer for their specific problems.

You've got to tell them what they're going to get, what is going to happen, and how they will feel as a result. But as I've said before, you can't communicate your value to your prospects until you recognize it yourself. So how do you recognize value?

It is not your job to convert people to your way of thinking. It is your job to speak your truth so that others may find theirs.

Start by asking yourself these questions:

- What are the benefits that I offer?
- What are the greatest results I can give people?
- What are the measurable improvements that I can bring to someone?
- How can THIS specific person who I'm speaking to benefit from my services?

If you look at the formula VALUE = DESIRABILITY divided by PRICE again, this makes perfect sense, and the most important piece of this to understand is: **When you clearly explain how your services will benefit someone (in ways that are really important to them), they will naturally desire them and value them more.**

There is a value hierarchy which applies to all goods and services. Here's how it works (in order from lowest to highest value):

- Commodity – If you're competing in the marketplace as a commodity, then you've got to have the lowest price. In other words, the cheapest price wins.

- Product – If you're competing as a product, someone might choose you over another brand because you're more familiar (someone might choose Crest toothpaste over Colgate, for example).

- Service – Someone might choose one acupuncturist over another simply because they provide a service that another acupuncturist does not, for example that acupuncturist takes their insurance. That practitioner provides a service that is unavailable at the other office. Unique benefits of the techniques or approaches aren't considered in the decision.

* Experience – Nordstrom department stores and Apple computers have created an "experience" in their stores. They offer more than just products and services, they offer a "feeling" that people want more of.

* Transformation – Transformation is the highest level of value. It involves offering a way to not just improve the life that someone is living, but to help them grow and evolve as a person.

Keep in mind, though, it's not the transformation itself that people want (offering that you provide "predictable transformation" would be too tangible). It's what the transformation enables in their life that's important; the deeper benefit behind the transformation. So, you need to figure out how to communicate how you transform peoples' lives.

One great way to illustrate the transformative potential of working with you is to have specific and detailed testimonials from your patients that tell the story of their struggles, journeys, and results. Instead of asking patients for a "review" or a "testimonial" consider asking them to share their "healing journey" in a review. Shifting that language helps to inspire them to leave a review that is more of a story of transformation, which is much more powerful. Everyone wants transformation.

If you can communicate concretely HOW you will transform someone's life and then deliver on it, you will be flooded with more business than you can handle!

Above all, seek to understand your current and potential patients. Find out what their frustrations, fears and challenges are. Think about what keeps them awake at night. Become totally passionate about their problems and embark on a crusade to solve them. Clearly communicate exactly how you will do this for them, and your practice will explode.

Taking it a step further – making sure it's in alignment with YOU

Now we are going to take it a step further. I want you to distinguish yourself from everyone else: What is unique about who you are, what you stand for, and what you do?

Remember, in order for you to stand out, and for people to "get" you, you've got to be real. You're communicating with humans, so be human! The norm is for acupuncturists to hide themselves behind facts or studies or bland statements, or even worse - jargon. They're meaningless. It's the wrong bait. What people are really looking for is human connection.

It's easier to rattle off jargon, but facts alone are not enough. They don't help you resonate unless they have an emotional impact. This doesn't mean that you should abandon facts entirely. Use plenty of facts, but accompany them with humanity.

Examples of humanless/sterile messages:

> *"Our clinic is the most reliable partner in your healthcare team, offering the best in quality and customer service to give you the best care we can."*

> *"Our clinic has more than 5 talented professionals dedicated to maximizing your results and experience."*

> *"Our clinic enriches lives with superior services at exceptional prices."*

> *"Our clinic empowers people, athletes, moms, and kids to reach heights they may have thought unreachable".*

Communicating only the detailed specifications of a product or service isn't enough. If two products have the same features, the one that appeals to an emotional need or creates a connection will be chosen.

So, what's the trick? Be somebody – yourself! Humans are social animals, and we're wired to interact. It's not the THING, it's the WHO associated with the thing. Think about artists - can you name a painting by Jackson Pollock, Picasso, or Norman Rockwell? For most of us, the answer is no, but we do know the ARTIST – the person, not the thing.

It's all about emotional connection. If you were looking at two identical offers, you would choose to buy or work with the one that you felt most connected to. How can you show people that haven't yet met you in person that you're willing to connect and really show up and hold space for them - that you're a real person? You must acknowledge that your potential patients need to connect with you as well as your medicine. It's not about trumpeting how great you are – it's about facilitating connection between you and your patients.

You may think, "I'm not that special" or "I just got out of school" or "I'm boring", and you don't want to come off as vain or conceited. But it's not bragging or vain or conceited to let yourself be seen a little bit. We're all here to contribute something unique. You have a special gift, you can make a difference, you can touch others' lives in a special way, and you can make the world a better place. You are UNIQUE.

Be uniquely you

In my area, there are a TON of acupuncturists. In fact, there is one RIGHT next door to my office! There is another one, who was actually my aaahmazing Basic Theory professor in grad school, just a few blocks away! I used to feel so self-conscious that people who could have been seeing him were seeing me, a newbie, instead, and driving right past his office to do so. I had to realize that regardless of my experience level, I had my own strengths. I had a lot to offer. The same is true of you, my friend.

You might have thought to yourself at some point, but aren't there already too many acupuncturists? Who am I, what do I know, how can I compete with those people who've been in practice for years? Well, what if Adele had said, "But doesn't the world have enough singers?" What if your favorite yoga studio said, "Does the world really need another yoga studio?" You've got to think about all of the goodness we would all miss out on if anyone stopped at the thought, hasn't it been done already?

"If you want the magical
formula for creating
a successful business,
it's actually you."

— Heather Nichols

There never has been and never will be another you. Only you can offer the services you do. We all do acupuncture, but we do it a little differently. You have a unique combination of experiences, interests, skills, talent, and personality. Only you can offer the exact combination of information, style of acupuncture, Qi, and communication that makes you so uniquely you. Truly know and believe you have great value. Then, others will know and appreciate what you have to offer.

You have a purpose - a very special gift that only you can bring to the world. So, when you do what you love, you are bringing the world something that it doesn't already have: your ideas. Your passion. Your touch. Your voice. The world really does want what you've got, and we're waiting for you to bring it to us.

The best way to be unique is to be authentic. Don't try to be unique. Just be authentic. I want you to embrace your story and your uniqueness. If you revel in it, expand on it, and use it to your advantage, you will be able to truly and deeply reach and help more people.

> Most of us acupuncturists become acupuncturists because we wanted meaning, connection, to touch lives. So why don't we bring those things into our marketing?

Exercise: Craft your bio. Tell it like a STORY, with a main character we can relate to, NOT just a list of facts. Think about the story of how you met your spouse. There's a quick version and the longer version, the funny version and the tragic version. Even if you're not married, you have other examples: stories that have been tested with different audiences repeatedly. Stories that have had certain elements tried and discarded, and other elements massaged and tweaked for maximum effect and the enjoyment of the listener. Do the same kind of thing with the story you're telling about yourself on your "about" page. Does it truly capture who you are, your passion, and all you have to offer? Does it show people that you're able to connect?

_____

_____

_____

_____

Next, let's pull it all together to hone in on your message.

Answer these 5 questions. Keep in mind your answers to all the previous exercises you've done in the book so far – your target patient and deeper benefits and your own story and strengths – so that you're thinking more specifically and in-depth about the many benefits that you provide. Take a look at everything you've written and then answer these:

1. What main problem does your service solve for your target patient (or one of your target markets)?

    _____

    _____

2. When someone (from that target market) uses your services, what are the implications for them in their life? Describe their needs and the positive results your services provide in detail.

    _____

    _____

3. What are you most proud of about your practice or service, and what makes you unique?

    _____

    _____

4. What do your clients really want?

    _____

    _____

5. Fill in these blanks:

    Get <u>acupuncture</u> so that you can

    _____

Now take the above sentence a step further:

You are _____ you want

_____ so that you can _____

Now take the above sentence a step further:

You are _____ you want

_____ so that you can _____

even if_____

For example: *You're a working mom, and you want to have more energy so that you can feel less overwhelmed and more present with your family, even if you feel like you have no time for self-care.*

Or: *You've suffered from bloating for years, and you've tried all the diets. You want to resolve your digestive issues so that you can go out to dinner without constantly worrying about locating the closest restroom. We can help, even if you've already tried everything.*

Or: *You're training for a marathon, and you want to prevent injury and support your endurance so that you can run without pain, even if you wonder if you're maybe a little too old to be running marathons.*

Once you've answered these questions and had some fun playing around with the fill-in-the-blank exercises, you will begin to see more clearly what a really great communication strategy and compelling message looks like for you and your target patients. Way to go!

Apply this message to all of your marketing efforts to make them effective at actually getting peoples' attention and inspiring them to action – especially on your website, and any flyers or ads that you may create. We'll talk more about key marketing mediums next.

Make yourself easy to "get"
and to talk about.

Chapter 10

Marketing is Like Gardening: Develop your Green Thumb

Now that you've started developing your message, and you know some of the deeper, specific, more compelling benefits of your services, the next step is to get that message out to the world.

Think of yourself as a gardener, and your practice as the garden.

To help drive home the benefit of taking a "gardener" approach to marketing, imagine instead for a moment that you're a hunter-gatherer who forages for meals. You go out into the world hungry, hoping to stumble upon things you can eat. You'll eat pretty much anything edible. Maybe you stumble onto a raspberry bush, so you get to eat a bunch of berries, which is great. But when you go back to the bush the next month, you don't know what will be there, if someone else ate them, or if it's been raining enough to nurture them – you're at the whim of nature as a hunger-gatherer.

Now, imagine you're a gardener. You walk out to your greenhouse, where you've learned to be quite a talented tomato and avocado grower. At first, it was a little challenging as you figured out exactly how much sunlight and water and room they needed. Over time, you got the hang of it, and now you have a dependable and delightful source of avocados and tomatoes that you love. Sometimes, you'll still eat some wild berries if you stumble upon them during your morning walk, but you don't have to go out searching or worrying. You've got a healthy and delicious source of sustenance you can count on.

One of the biggest mistakes that acupuncturists make is foraging or scavenging instead of actively cultivating their garden. Most acupuncturists take the "hunter-gatherer" approach to attracting patients: they try to drum up patients instantly, wandering around, trying various things and desperately looking various places, hoping to find patients they can treat ASAP. The problems with this are obvious: they're at the whim of nature, and they pretty much have to take whatever they get. At best, this method of sustenance is cyclical, but often frustrating.

The better way to go is to plant your own seeds as a proactive gardener. You won't have to go out foraging for whatever's out there, instead growing your own reliable, predictable sustenance that *you* like.

If you maintain and nourish those seeds, you can harvest them when the time is right. It's not instant gratification, but it's an investment in your future. I think of the "seeds" you plant as the various ways you start relationships with potential patients and let them know you're there, and I think of "fertilizing" your garden as your ability to foster the trust, connection, and relationship with those potential patients - to keep in touch and to reside in the "front of mind" space. Because otherwise life gets in the way. You may be referred to someone who would love to come in for your services, but for any number of reasons they're unable to commit in that moment. That's life. But, if you have some systems in place where you can keep in touch with that person through non-spammy emails, social media, or your website, when your potential patient is ready, YOU are the one who comes to their mind. You can't rely on the customer to remember you, or to keep your business card, or to keep your communication open. It's your responsibility to keep in touch. That's what I mean by fertilizing your garden.

The other problem with scavenging instead of gardening is that you rely solely on picking the low-hanging fruit that happens to be available. Most acupuncturists are doing this with their marketing because their messages are vague, general, and the same as everyone else's: "Try acupuncture!" or "I'm an acupuncturist!" or "Acupuncture works!" They're not educating people about how they can specifically help them, and they're not speaking their language, resonating with them or drawing them in. They're missing an opportunity to turn someone who didn't have acupuncture on their radar at all into someone who is eager to try acupuncture.

Most acupuncturists, by keeping their messages vague and general, are just trying to find the people - or worse, waiting around for people to find them - who already know they want acupuncture. So, most acupuncturists are fishing out of the same small pond.

We've got to reach people who didn't even know about acupuncture or that it could help them, and turn them into people who are excited to get your services. You've got to reach them and educate them and speak to them in their language. This is how we grow the size of our pond or reach past the low-hanging fruit, or sow a large field of potential patients clamoring for our services. This is how we grow demand for acupuncture. This is how we educate people about acupuncture. This is how we elevate or profession. This is how we show the world that we mean business.

If you honestly think that you can get all you can out of your career by sitting back and waiting for the world to seek YOU out, then you're delusional. Sorry, tough love, but true. It's just as likely as the apple tree chasing down the forager; it just doesn't happen that way. But this is exactly what you're doing if your marketing message is vague, general, confusing, or all about you, and your marketing efforts are disorganized, short-sighted and lacking strategy.

All you have to do is turn on some systems or strategies that will get your message that you've developed in the previous chapter out there, and then keep in touch with potential patients in a manner that respects them, adds value and cultivates their trust in and connection with you. And when they're ready, you're right there to serve them. I think of this as planting seeds and fertilizing your garden patch.

Sowing seeds

The seeds are the little messages that get planted into the world. They represent various ways in which people might be introduced to you and your work; the possibility that you might be able to help them. It's the beginning of a client's relationship with you.

Let's talk about some of the different seeds you can plant.

Seeds:

- Search engine referrals
- Blog posts
- Video blogs, Facebook lives or Youtube videos
- Building relationships with doctors and other healthcare professionals
- Direct-to consumer-ads (Google ads, Facebook ads, or flyers)

When you focus on getting good at one thing at a time, that's when the breakthroughs happen. That's when you reach the tipping point.

Keep-in-touch plan:

- Social media
- Email

Hub:

- Your website

Aside from search engine referrals via SEO, a practice that everyone should harness which I'll talk more about later, I recommend picking one type of seed from the list above to start, and sticking with it consistently. You don't need to do "all the things." That's a recipe for burnout – it will leave you overwhelmed, and will likely create consistency issues, resulting in poor outcomes. It's like the amateur acupuncturist who puts in way too many needles, throwing ALL THE THINGS at the problem, hoping one of them does the trick. This is not an effective way to treat, nor is it an effective way to grow a business. You need to have a diagnosis, process, and plan. Similarly, all the things do not lead to all the patients; that will burn you out. While it can be a good idea to try out each of the seed strategies for a short time in the beginning as a way to experiment and determine the best course for you, I recommend, after brief experimentation, picking one seed strategy to stick with consistently.

Let's say you decide you're going to blog regularly. It will get easier after doing it several times - you'll develop systems around it as well as traction and momentum. Create a plan, put it into your schedule, and stick with it. It's far easier and less overwhelming to pick one seed strategy, develop systems for it, and do it consistently and efficiently.

This is what I chose: I blogged once a month for the first two years of my practice. Each blog post took me many hours at first, and then I got better and faster at it. I got better at sourcing my ideas and inspiration, writing headlines, and letting my own beliefs and approaches flow onto the page more naturally. Now, I can write a blog post in about an hour. It feels good to share my wisdom with the world and help people.

This approach helped me get my website to page one of Google within a year of graduating. But moreover, it also showed people who came to my website that I'm an expert. It showed people that I have a lot to offer, that my approach is accessible and methodical, and that they can trust me. It helps people to find me (via Google), and then once they've landed on my website, it helps them to trust me and want to work with me.

But blogging isn't for everyone, and a different type of "seed" may feel more natural to you. You might decide you hate writing, and that it's easier, faster, and more natural for you to put together a 5-minute video blog. You might decide you'd rather spend your time developing relationships with doctors who will hopefully refer to you. That's why I give you several different options for your seed strategy. I urge you to pick the one that feels most natural to you, because that's the one that you'll stick with consistently. Even if your seed of choice is developing relationships with other health professionals, that still takes consistency. Don't just approach a doctor once and then be bummed that he/she never refers a patient to you. You've got to follow up. Just like with blogging, it takes consistently doing it over time to see the results.

You may also decide that you'd rather spend money than time on planting seeds. Maybe you don't like writing or video blogs or networking, and you find it easier and more comfortable to pay for ads, sit back, and let them do the work for you. That's fine, too. This method also takes consistency, however, because there is a learning curve to figuring out what ads resonate with and convert patients. If you choose to go the advertising route, make sure that you're doing it in a way that allows you to track the results - the pay-off of your investment. That way, you're not just hemorrhaging cash on ads, and you know that your money is being wisely invested in a way that translates to more patients. Look at the data of your results and measure your progress. Stick with it and tweak your ads until the data shows you're getting good results. Just like all the seeds, it takes time.

I recommend picking your seed and sticking with it consistently over time. Look at the list above and ask yourself - what feels most natural and easiest to me? The one that comes the easiest to you will be the one that you are able to stick with more consistently. And consistency is key.

Please notice what's *not* listed as a "seed":

- Networking groups
- Health fairs
- Social media
- Word of mouth referrals
- Results
- Getting involved in the community

I don't consider those "seeds" for a few reasons.

Many people can say that networking groups like BNI are effective for them, and that they helped to attract more people to their practice. But as soon as they leave the group, stop paying their dues, and stop being active, the benefits fall away. It's not a great long-term game.

Health fairs are generally not an efficient use of your time. Sure, when I used to do the farmers market in my neighborhood, I'd get some patients signed up. But it took hours and hours of my time (grueling time for me as an introvert who wanted to shrivel up and die at the fact that I was putting myself out there like that). And again, once you stop doing health fairs, they stop being beneficial for you.

I put social media in the "keep in touch" category, instead of the "seed" category because, while social media might help bring in new patients, they are the exception, not the rule. And I try to only recommend strategies that can be predictably and reliably replicated to produce successful results. Even for acupuncturists who have followings of more than 10K followers, social media primarily helps to fill cancellations; it doesn't lead to a steady and reliable source of new patients. It serves better as a way to stay connected with people and remind them that you're there. But for the amount of time and effort it takes to create an effective social media presence, I frankly just don't think it's worth it. It also stops working for you when you stop doing it, so it's not a great long-term strategy. Now if you love it and it fills you up, then you will be the exception to this rule, and by all means my friend, go for it; do it with consistency and fervor and love. But for the vast majority of us, I'd wager to say that maintaining a consistent social media presence can feel draining rather than empowering.

Word-of-mouth referrals are not a "strategy." They are something that should naturally occur in your clinic as a result of you delivering excellent care. Everyone's plan should be to provide great care and results, and to generate word-of-mouth referrals organically and naturally. It doesn't feel good for me to ask for them - that feels cheesy and awkward. I prefer to inspire them rather than ask for or incentivize them.

The above concept is linked to the next item on the list – results. Despite how often people tout this as a "strategy," I don't consider "just get great results" to be a marketing strategy. Get great results, absolutely. But this is customer service; it's a baseline. It's a bare minimum. Sitting and waiting for people to refer to you is not a proactive, empowered way to build your practice. Eventually, once you've been in practice a long time and have a very large group of people who've experienced your care, you might be able to ride on word-of-mouth referrals and results. But until you've grown your patient list enough, it's not going to grow your patient base very quickly. Only a fraction of people who get referred to you actually take action and come in, so you need a very large number of people talking about you in order for it to move the needle on your practice.

Getting involved in the community is a great thing to do. Going back to our hunter-gatherer vs gardening example, community involvement is great in that it is more like gardening than "foraging" because it can be a long term approach and different than trying to convince strangers you just met that they need to book an appointment with you (which just makes me feel weird. That would be like walking up to a stranger at the bar and saying, "Will you marry me?" Like, what? Who are you and why should I trust you? It just doesn't work that way. I'm an introvert, and I'm not just going to introduce myself to strangers or presume to boss them around and tell them what to do or promote myself like that. No way, that's just not how I am. So, when business coaches tell acupuncturists to talk to strangers and to start a conversation in some slick way with some weird pick-up line about the work you do, it makes me cringe.) Getting authentically involved in your community is different, because they're not strangers, and therefore does fall more towards being a gardening "seed." It doesn't involve some slick conversation. It just involves you being yourself and developing relationships over time, which I can totally get behind.

But I still don't think this is really a strategy. I think it's just life, and it just happens. Talk to people, be a person, do things you're interested in, and let people know you're an acupuncturist, because that's a huge part of who you are. You don't need a marketing teacher to tell you to live your life or talk to people. You don't need a slick line, you don't need a salesy and gimmicky elevator pitch, because that just hurts trust. So please just develop sincere and genuine relationships with people. That is key to success, and you don't need a business teacher telling you how to do that. You just need to be yourself.

Community involvement should happen organically, otherwise you won't stick with it and be consistent, and it won't really amount to much. Let's say you brainstormed ways you could get involved in your community, and you decided you should go to more yoga classes. Great. But if you don't stick with it over time because it's not actually an interest or passion of yours, it won't work to cultivate relationships of trust. Don't go to a random yoga class here and there and then pat yourself on the back because you're "marketing" because that sporadic approach probably won't amount to much. If you're going to do it, commit to it. If there's something you've been really wanting to do or get involved in, and if starting to view it as also a good business decision will be the kick in the pants you need to get you to chase your dreams, then do it! And if you have any ideas for ways to get involved that will also be personally fulfilling for you, write them down here:

_____

_____

_____

_____

I'll bet that in life, most people who meet you tend to automatically trust and like you, and they want to work with you. What really helps grow your practice is when you can expand *that* know-like-trust to be present for not just the people that you meet in real life, but for people who find you online or through your marketing "seeds," too. *That's* the key to attracting more patients with ease. Just like with meeting people in real life, it's not about being gimmicky or coming up with some slick line. It's actually being a genuine person.

So, hopefully, I've made it clear why the list of possible "seeds" includes certain activities and excludes others. Generally, it's because the best "seeds" are replicable for the vast majority of us, and when done consistently for a period of time, will continue working for us well into the future once they are stopped.

Exercise: Decide which seed strategy you'd like to focus on. Think about your past or current marketing efforts and ask yourself: what kind of seeds have I planted in the past? Have I been consistent with any of them? What has worked well and felt natural for me? Can I become more consistent with it moving forward? Look at the list of possible "seeds," and make notes of which "seeds" you're going to get better and more consistent at planting and nurturing.

_____

_____

_____

_____

"Be yourself no matter what. Some will adore you and some will hate everything about you. But who cares? It's your life. Make the most out of it."

~ Unknown

Build your authority

When you are sowing your seeds and nourishing your garden, it's important to realize that your potential patients are always asking themselves, "Can I trust this person, and can they help me?"

Make it really easy for people to trust you by showing that you're an *authority*. How do you do that? The letters behind your name aren't enough, sorry. You've got to share some of your knowledge. Let them experience it and appreciate it and think, *"Wow, this person knows helpful things! I trust their opinion and perspective."*

You're someone who has great information and expertise, and a *process* for treating so many conditions. You're so much more than just a slinger of needles. You're an authority with a unique perspective and approach. Don't let yourself be merely a commodity by failing to let people see your expertise.

What do I mean by "commodity"? Think of gas in your car, which is a commodity - you'll always go to the gas station with the lowest price, right? You wouldn't pay more for gas from a different gas station nearby. All gas is basically the same, and all you care about is price. That's what makes it a commodity.

Do you want your patients to *only* care about your price? No. You want them to choose you because they resonate with you, and because of your unique experience and perspective, and because they trust you. They believe that you can help them. That's what I think of as your "authority" – they trust you know what you're doing and can help them.

You want people who are complete strangers to you to land on your website and think, *this person seems to know what they're talking about. It's clear that they get me and my problem, and I think they might be able to help me! Omg, there's hope for me! Where do I sign up?*

Show that you're an expert with answers. There are many ways to do this:

1. By having condition-specific pages on your website where you discuss those conditions, how you can help, and what people can expect.
2. By having condition-specific testimonials and reviews.
3. By having a blog or vlog (video blog) where you give helpful + actionable information on how people can improve their problem.
4. By giving talks at local events.
5. By building referral relationships with doctors.

The first two are a must-do. For #3 – 5, choose at least one that feels good, easy, and in alignment for you, and start there.

Building your authority while creating connections and tapping into service in ways that are meaningful to your ideal patients' deeper needs and desires - this is the recipe for success in attracting patients.

Key to this is creating regular content that displays your expertise and knowledge. AND it has to be helpful. Whether this is giving live talks, blogging, FB live videos, or YouTube videos, you've got to be creating consistently original content, or creating a relationship with an established authority (a doctor or other health professional) whose referrals will build your authority for you by recommending you to patients.

The key is that, by showing that you are a trusted authority, potential patients will see you're an expert, trust you, and have even more clarity about how you can help them and what they have going on.

Choose the medium or avenue that feels best to you. Which one feels the most naturally aligned to you?

_____

_____

Next, consider your ideal patients. Where are they? Are they on social media? Are they not really hanging out on social media, and probably just Googling for answers? Are they not Googling for answers, but instead relying solely on their doctors' recommendations and referrals? Go to where your potential patients are, and give them what will resonate with them. As long as it also aligns with you.

If one of the strategies for sharing your authority doesn't jump out at you immediately, then I recommend feeling it out at first by trying a few. Write a couple blog posts, film a few videos, reach out to a few doctors, and see how it feels. Then, pick the one that feels the most naturally aligned with you, and stick with it. Know that it will feel awkward at first, and that with time and practice, it will get WAY easier. But perhaps one will feel slightly more natural than the other.

Focus on the LONG game

It's important to focus on the long game, not short-sighted flash-in-the-pan marketing tactics like health fairs, networking groups, telling strangers you meet about acupuncture, and ads offering huge discounts. Any strategies that are trying to get patients in the door right now, that don't have systems in place for long-term engagement, are harmful to the long game.

The real key to making marketing both effective and easy for yourself is to focus on creating systems and assets that build genuine connections with people. Build systems that will continue to work for you in the long run, bringing patients in the door without you having to do additional work. I recommend doing this by choosing one strategy to sow your "seeds" and building your authority, developing systems and schedules, and sticking with them consistently.

For example, I chose the seed and authority-building strategy of blogging. I created a system for it – a way of doing it that was repeatable - and a time in my schedule that "triggered" it to happen. I first brainstormed a list of topic ideas to write about over the year, and then every Tuesday in the early afternoon, I'd look at my list and write a blog post for the week. A system doesn't need to be high-tech or complex, it just means there is an event or time that "triggers" it to get done and a way of going about it that delivers the desired result consistently.

It's creating assets and systems so you don't have to be out there engaging constantly. Blog posts will still be out there in the internet working for you in the long run without you having to do more work - this turns blogging into a long-term asset. I can see (via Google Analytics) that my blog posts I wrote back in 2011 and 2012 are still going "viral," performing well on Google, and attracting thousands of people to my website each month. Doctors and other health professionals will continue to refer to you long into the future once a solid foundation of trust and mutual respect has been established, turning this relationship into a long-term asset.

The key is to focus on the long game. I know that when acupuncturists are just starting out, it can feel like "Ah, where is everybody?" You can feel a little panicked, like you need to get patients in the door ASAP. As a result, many acupuncturists focus on short-term flash-in-the-pan marketing strategies that take a lot of energy and don't actually work, rather than focusing on creating those long-term assets. That's to their huge disadvantage because they'll likely always be just treading water and never getting ahead if they don't focus on the long game.

So, please take a deep breath and focus on creating those long-term assets and systems that grow your practice. While these strategies may not get you patients in the door immediately, if you do them consistently, they will absolutely bring you a steady stream of loyal patients, starting in a few months and continuing into the future. The problem is, people stop executing these strategies because they think, "Well, I wrote a blog post and no one came in the door the next day." That's right - that's not how it works. People aren't going to come in the door the next day because they read your blog post, but over several months to a year of consistently doing it, it will very likely attract patients.

In the beginning especially, you will need to get patients in the door ASAP. I think the easiest way to do this is to write a brief, friendly, and personal email to everyone you know in your area announcing that you're open for new patients, sharing the specific types of patients and conditions you especially love to work with, and inviting people to come in and see you or refer or friend or reach out to you with questions. You could consider offering a limited-time discount, but it's a mistake to only focus on the discount without focusing on the value you offer by specifically describing the conditions you get results for and love to work with. You could also do the short-term "scavenging" strategy of introducing yourself to other businesses in your neighborhood and inviting them to come in and experience your care. However, you are making your life more difficult if you spend all your time on these short-term strategies while neglecting the long-term strategies. In a few months of consistently putting the long-term strategies to work for you, you will be able to let go of the short-term "scavenging" strategies and ride on the simple systems you've put into place.

You want to focus on doing what you love and treating patients, not constantly scavenging for patients. So, pick your seed strategy - that will be the way you contribute, connect, and show up to serve. When you stick with it and build it over time, it will continue working for you. As it continues to work for you, it will build upon itself, amplifying its effect for greater impact and reach. In order to accomplish this, though, you've got to focus on the long-game, not flash-in-the-pan stuff. We can be completely overwhelmed by all the marketing advice out there. "Oh, I have to do this, and that, and this." You don't have to do all the things; you have to pick the one that feels in alignment with you. Do it consistently and do it well, and create systems for doing it with ease.

With a consistent gardening strategy combined with a clear, resonant message that you developed in the previous chapters, you will become irresistible to the people you're meant to serve. And you won't have to spend a ton of time and energy worrying about "marketing." You'll just be consistently sowing your "seeds," and connecting with and serving people.

Set-it-and-forget-it marketing

I really want to plant the set-it-and-forget-it marketing idea in your head.

Lighthouses don't go running
all over the island looking
for boats to save; they just
stand there shining.

As acupuncturists who love our medicine and want to help people, we've sort of reluctantly found ourselves in the role of small-business owner, whose job is partly to get people in the door to benefit from our services. And it kind of sucks, right? That's not really how we want to be spending our time. I don't. I don't want to spend my time marketing; I want to be treating patients.

As a result, we are all weighing a calculation in our head. A calculation of energy, effort, time, cost, and emotional energy put into our marketing efforts weighed against the potential benefit and result of that input.

But from what I can tell, a lot of acupuncturists are weighing this calculation without knowing all the information. I think they are overestimating the effort required for a lot of types of marketing, specifically online marketing, and underestimating the results.

They overestimate the effort because they just assume it's really hard and confusing, and they underestimate the results because the results are usually not immediate. But here's the thing: Even though the results don't happen immediately, over time, that little bit of initial effort continues to work and work and work even more for you.

Most acupuncturists are instead doing things like networking groups, health fairs or discounts, because those might lead to an immediate inflow of patients. But they stop working for you once you stop putting the effort in, so it's a very short-sighted approach that keeps you on that hamster wheel. You have to constantly continue your marketing efforts, and it drains you and burns you out.

It's really frustrating for me to watch this when there is a much easier way. I call it set-it-and-forget-it marketing.

Here is my 4-step system for attracting patients on auto-pilot:

1. Build confidence, trust, and rapport in the intake process
2. Good SEO – so you show up exactly when people need you
3. A website that inspires people to sign up
4. An opt-in email funnel that takes the pressure off of people to book with you immediately and builds authority and connection.

The beauty of this 4-step system is that not only does it work, but it continues to work for you – that's why it's called "set-it-and-forget-it".

Step 1: Build confidence, trust, rapport, and referrals in the intake process. This is what makes people really want to do what you say, follow your advice, stick with your treatment plan, work with you, commit to their long-term care with you, and refer their friends and family. Most of the acupuncturists I mentor think that they're already doing this. And this is a wonderful thing about acupuncturists – the meaningful relationships we build with our patients. However, there are almost always three simple yet important pieces missing to their Intake: 1) listening very carefully for the "why" and the real issue beyond the chief complaint or their list of symptoms, and echoing this back to them so that they feel you hear and understand them; 2) asking the patient what they feel the solution may be – this is a coaching technique that helps inspire patients to take action and invest in their care; and 3) when giving them your recommendation, clearly linking with simple language your care to their big "why" and their desired result.

I think of learning the art of an effective intake as a prerequisite to learning about marketing, since marketing would be a waste of everyone's time and energy if you weren't able to engage and inspire those patients to stick around long enough to get results. Developing patient rapport and trust, and earning referrals in the initial intake is important. While subtle, it's not complicated, and once you make these few simple shifts in the intake process, it feels really good for both you and your patients.

The take home here is that your intake process must inspire confidence, rapport, referrals, and trust. The question to ask yourself is, on average, how many treatments are my patients coming to me for? If the number is lower than 8, and if you're often hearing, "Thank you very much, but I can't afford your services," then something's not quite working with your intake process. How often are people referring their family and friends to you after their initial visit with you? If that's not happening, then something is off with your intake. And that's good news, because this is really easy to change, and doing so can make a huge difference for your practice.

Step 2: The second pillar of set-it-and-forget marketing is being able to show up in the exact moment when your potential patients need you. How do you do this? With good SEO.

Google is an amazing referral source. Statistics show that 8 out of 10 people turn to Google first when seeking health info, and that 86% of internet users have searched for a health topic online. In this day in age, we tend to trust Google the most when it comes to recommendations. We'll click on a link because Google recommended it. And Google tries really hard to earn and maintain this trust, because all those viewers and users lead to advertising revenue for them.

So, people trust and use Google, as you probably do. Do you search for answers on Google? I do. But the real power of Google and good SEO is in perfect timing. When someone searches for you - say they search acupuncture back pain Denver - they are actively looking for a solution to a problem. They're actually looking for you, meaning that they're usually ready to take action. If you show up in that EXACT moment, that's powerful. So much more powerful than, say, a random social media post that appears when people aren't actively looking for a solution - so they ignore it. This is an amazing service to provide. You can show up exactly when people need you and are ready to take action, and light the way for them. Show them the path. Let them know you understand them, and that you can lead them.

And it's really simple to do it yourself. It may take about 3 – 4 hours of your time to implement all the steps, and once that's done, it's done. You set it and forget it. It doesn't happen overnight; it takes a bit of time. You'll watch yourself slowly rise in SEO ranking. Usually it takes about 4-6 weeks after implementation for people to see their page rank rise and notice that more people are being referred from the Internet.

It's one of the best "seeds" you can plant because it's a set-it-and-forget-it seed. It's a constant referral source. It gets people to your website when they are in need of your services. They know they need your services, and are actively looking for you. They're ready to take action, but only with the help of a source that people trust. It's a great referral source to your website.

This leads us to the 3rd step.

Step 3: Your website. You don't just need a website; you need a website that works for you (for free) by answering the questions people most want to know and inspiring them to take action and schedule an appointment with you. If you already have a website, ask yourself - what do people think when they land on your website? Does it resonate with them? Are they scheduling with you? Does it inspire trust, confidence, connection, and action? Or do most people click away? You can measure this with your bounce rate in Google Analytics (which is free), by the way.

Most acupuncture websites are all pretty similar, and they're all making the same mistakes. They aren't patient-centric. They're vague, focusing only on the practitioner and their modalities, or tools. It's ironic, because in our medicine, our care is so patient-focused. But we can lose that when it comes to our marketing. Typically, we start focusing all on ourselves, instead of what the patients care about and need to hear from you the most. I think we have good intentions, we just don't know what else to say, so we say what we know already – and that's usually all about our medicine and ourselves.

People need to know your story and what you stand for, but more than that, they need to know what you can do for them and why they should trust you. Your website needs to be the hub for that, and it needs to clearly and immediately provide a sense of what you're about.

There's a lot to this, but here's a quick tip: People don't care about your tools (needles, moxa, herbs). They care about your results. They care about how likely you are to have the solution to their problem. If you have a leaky toilet, and you go to a plumber's website, and they talk all about their pipe-wrench and socket-wrench, you're lost and you don't care. You want them to say, "Leaky toilet? We've got your back."

Too many acupuncturists' websites talk all about moxa and cupping and gua sha and tui na and estim – they list those as their services. News flash: those are not the services you provide. Those are your tools. And yes, they're cool tools (cooler than a socket-wrench in my opinion), but the services you provide are WAY more amazing than that. You help people start families, you relieve peoples' pain, you help people become free from anxiety, and the list goes on. These are amazing services! So, make sure you're telling people what you really do, and what they really care about.

But here's the thing: I know that's a hard task because acupuncture is amazing at so many things, and the possibilities are endless. And here's the real kicker: You can't just copy someone else's website, or someone else's anything. It's got to come from your heart.

Just as we can't throw some cookie-cutter version of acupuncture points at a problem, but have to start with D&D (differential diagnosis), the same goes for finding your best marketing message. The same set of acupuncture points won't work for every headache. And the same website or ad copy won't work for every acupuncturist. You've got to walk through a simple, yet thorough process first, kind of like our D&D, to make sure you're hitting the mark.

It takes some time, soul-searching, and articulating things that can be hard to articulate. Go back to that marketing message you developed in the previous chapter, and make sure that's on your website. If you did those exercises for more than one target audience and target patient, and you have more than one message, fine! Great! Make sure they're all on your website in places that make sense – most likely on condition-specific pages. And once you do? It's done. You can set it and forget it. And then, people who land on your website will be much more likely to hit the "schedule now" button.

This brings us to the 4th pillar.

Step 4: An opt-in email funnel that takes the pressure off people to book with you immediately, allowing you to further build authority and connection.

But what if they still aren't quite ready to hit the schedule now button? Let's take the pressure off of people. They just met you. They landed on your website. You don't just walk up to someone in a bar and say, "Want to have dinner with me?" or, remember that Top Gun line, "Take me to bed or lose me forever"? Do you want to say, "Hi I'm Katie, an acupuncturist, schedule now or lose me forever"?

No, I don't want to pressure people. Personally, I want to empower and inspire people. You should absolutely have online scheduling. And encourage people to schedule an appointment with you or to schedule a free initial consult or discovery call with you.

But you can also encourage people to get to know you, your solutions, philosophy, and approach a little better with a free opt-in email series. This allows you to build better connection, confidence, and trust over time. And maybe, after that series, they'll be far more ready and excited to schedule and work with you, regardless of your prices.

Ask yourself what you could offer potential patients that would be really interesting and compelling for them, and maybe even get them a quick win towards their desired result – it could be your top 10 tips for reducing anxiety, for example, if anxiety is one of your target markets. One helpful tip for figuring this out is to look at what some of your most popular blog posts are and ask yourself if you could make a quick worksheet based on them. I like short, concise PDFs that give patients a quick win. You can design a professional-looking PDF for free on Canva.com. This will be your "lead magnet" for your email funnel.

Then, you can set up your email list and opt-in form in an email service such as Mailchimp or ConvertKit (I use Convertkit personally, but Mailchimp is good because, if you have fewer than 1000 subscribers, it's free). Display the opt-in form in relevant areas on your website, and write a handful of emails that are related to the topic of your lead magnet. Continue to deliver more helpful information with a series of emails that will get automatically sent through your email service provider. Here's how I like to structure my email series:

1. Deliver the lead magnet that they requested

2. Introduce yourself and your work (in a way that specifically relates to the lead magnet topic, if possible)

3. Share a testimonial that's related to the lead magnet topic

4. Invite them to work with you and schedule an appointment

5. Add them to your regular email list, so in the future, they receive your newsletter emails as a reminder of the ways you can help them

You can set this email series up for free, but that's not the best part. The best part is that it's AUTOMATIC. Once it's set up, you don't have to do anything. It just works in the background, regardless of what you're doing. You write those emails once, and then you're done. They get sent automatically whenever someone signs up from your website. You set it and forget it.

So, those are the 4 crucial steps. First, you need an intake process that inspires trust, confidence, action, and referrals. Then, you need SEO so you get referrals from Google, which is a hugely trusted source these days. Next, you need a website that inspires people to want to work with you. Finally, you need an email series that takes the pressure off and builds connection and trust. These are all set-it-and-forget-it marketing systems. You do the work once, and they go on working for you without you having to do anything.

Stop expecting people to automatically know that they need acupuncture, and that you can help them. Don't expect them to choose you when they don't know anything about you or how you can help them. If you haven't displayed any reason to trust you besides having an L.Ac. behind your name, then why should they choose you?

Start expecting to show up, share value, and build relationships. The great news? These days, you can share your value and your truth while building relationships with the set-it-and-forget-marketing systems I reviewed for you. This is what the busy acupuncture clinics are doing to attract patients on autopilot.

This is how you get out of the never-ending, constantly-need-to-do-marketing trap. You can get a steady stream of patients to your practice, and focus on doing what you love – practicing your medicine and assisting with peoples' healing journeys.

Your website is the hub of your garden

The best place to start? With your hub. The thing that will be central to all of it - your website.

It's your hub because that's where everyone will go no matter how they learned about you. It's where they go to get scheduled.

Even when someone hears about you from a doctor or personal recommendation, the first thing they'll do is check out your website. Make sure it's working for you.

You need it to:

- Clearly convey the benefits of working with you

- Act as a front desk person that can 24/7 answer frequently asked questions about your location, prices, hours, services, and what to expect

- Collect email addresses with an opt-in form and lead magnet

- Display your expertise and build your authority and trust

What does your website say currently? Most websites and marketing start with "me-ness". It's important that people know something about you and your company, but put the bulk of that on a secondary page, and focus on a message that resonates with your market instead.

When trying to connect with current or potential patients, you have to remember that it's not ALL about you. People detest arrogance and self-centeredness. You know the feeling of going to a party and being cornered by a dreadful, self-centered know-it-all who talks all about himself and his own interests, how cool he is, and etc., while you're looking for any opportunity to escape. Why is that? It's because the conversation doesn't INCLUDE you, your ideas, or your perspective. Self-centered people don't connect. No one wants to date, work with, or talk with someone like that, so why is marketing rife with self-centered content?

As a healthcare practitioner, it's easy to feel like our education, our services, and our expertise should be the most important thing. We may even think, "I'm their hero, here to save them from their helplessness and ignorance. If they only knew what I know, the world would be a better place." But if we present ourselves like that and make it all about us, our services, and our knowledge, then we become the self-centered know-it-all at the party, and people will want to flee.

Instead, let's embrace humility and deference to our patients' needs. Let's market from a shared place of understanding. Make it about them. Our patient (or potential patient) is the hero. So, what's our role, then? We are the mentor. We're Yoda, not Luke Skywalker.

Our patients are the ones who will do the heavy lifting to reach their objectives. We're simply one voice helping them get unstuck as they make their journey. As mentor, our role is to give the hero guidance, confidence, insight, advice, and an acupuncture treatment that will harness their own body's healing ability. They're going to actually do the work.

Ensuring that we embrace the role of mentor with even our website and marketing strategies will ensure that we come from a place of humility. This approach will help us gain resonance with our current and potential patients. I recommend taking a look at your website and asking yourself where you're shining the light – on yourself and your clinic, or on the patient? Focusing on the patient will ensure that when the right person reads your message, they'll say to themselves, "That's me, she gets me! That's totally what I'm looking for!" It is the difference between "That looks interesting" and "I'm definitely getting that!".

The way to get people to say "That's me!" is to spend the time thinking about your patients and asking the right questions so that you can hone in on what's really going on in their world, the deeper reasons and frustrations that brought them to you, and the deeper results and desires they are looking for as an outcome of working with you, as you did in the previous chapter. I encourage you to revisit those exercises again and again. They're huge. Every time I re-do the exercise, I get something even better, deeper, and truer.

To better connect with your potential patients, focus on adding value, and avoid trying to "sell" them your services. Instead, educate them, explain the benefits of your solution, and show them how you can solve their problems. The easiest way to do this is by adding condition-specific pages on your website. Your services are the results of your care, and you need to highlight those.

Go back to the previous chapter and look at the target audiences you developed, and then make sure you have a dedicated page on your website for each of those audiences - a page that speaks directly to them. Do you love working with fertility? Make sure you have a fertility page on your website. Work a lot with back pain? Make sure you have a page specifically for that on your website. Want to work with IBS and digestive issues more? Dedicate a page of your website to it.

It's not only good for SEO, it will make people trust you more. After landing on your website and thinking, "Am I in the right place, can this person help me?" they'll see that specific page that's written just for them and their problem – and they'll know they ARE in the right place.

Exercise: Maybe you have some ideas coming up now for tweaks you'd like to make to your website. Make note of those here:

_____

_____

_____

_____

Fertilizing your garden

Email marketing and social media are two vital ways to keep in touch and nurture your working relationships. They allow you to stay connected with your patients and potential patients, to continue to cultivate trust, and to remind them that you're there and would love to help them, their friends, and their families while delivering further value to your community. Here are some ideas of things you can provide through email and/or social media:

- General or seasonal health tips

- Success stories

- Inspirational quotes

- Relevant insights from your own life

- Recommended reading

- Favorite healthy recipes or resources

- Other inspirational and motivational content

Email is more effective than social media. Social media "algorithms" purposefully limit your content to a fraction of your audience, but emailing allows you to bypass the algorithm and go straight to their inbox. Emailing your patients and potential patients regularly and consistently reminds them that you're there for them, while at the same time educating and inspiring them in a way that adds value. The best part is that it doesn't take much time at all to send out regular emails once you've got your system set up.

Here are some tips for getting started.

Step 1: Build your email list.

Collect your patients' email addresses. The easiest way to do this is to ask for this on their intake paperwork (be sure to get their permission before putting them on your regular mailing list). If you don't have email addresses for your current patients, be sure to ask them.

Put an email opt-in box on your website to capture the emails of potential patients, and inform them of what they should expect in their inboxes, while assuring them you won't sell or share their email info with any other parties. I recommend trading some valuable information in exchange for email addresses, such as a free report on a common health challenge that you treat, as we talked about before: the "lead magnet".

Step 2: Subscribe to an email marketing service

I like mailchimp.com or convertkit.com, but there are many other options available online. An email marketing service will let you transfer your email addresses from your database into an online account. From there, you can categorize them into various lists, choose from graphic templates to create professionally designed emails, monitor all of your email marketing statistics, and more. An email service also does two other important things: 1) it makes you far less likely to end up in the spam folder when emailing a large group, and 2) it allows people to choose to "unsubscribe" from your emails, which you are required to do by law if you are regularly emailing a large group for commercial purposes. So, you definitely need to use an email marketing service.

Step 3: Decide on a frequency

Decide how often you are going to contact your list. Is it once a week, once a month, or once a quarter? I recommend once or twice a month – just enough to remain top-of-mind, and not too much to overwhelm them. Pick your frequency and stick with it so that your readers know what to expect. Schedule an hour of time to write it and get it sent out – go ahead and schedule this into your calendar at whatever frequency you decided for the whole year. In general, the best time to send an email is in the early afternoon on a Tuesday or Wednesday.

Step 4: Don't take unsubscribes personally!

When you start emailing your audience on a regular basis, you're going to get some unsubscribes. Even people who still visit you regularly might opt-out of your email list. Remember, it's not about you. If someone doesn't want to receive emails from you any longer, it's probably because they don't have the time to read them, or they just try to unsubscribe from everything and keep their inbox lean – totally understandable, in my opinion.

If you're getting a lot of opt-outs, however, you might be sending out too many emails that are either: 1) not relevant to what your audience cares about, 2) going out too frequently, or 3) too self-serving and "promotional". Send relevant emails that are short, concise, and informative, and you'll develop a following that is eager to open your emails.

Step 5: Be consistent!

People will get used to receiving your emails, and if your messages are valuable and beneficial to them, they'll actually miss them when they don't get them!

If you do these two things, 1) hone your website so it speaks directly to your potential patients while also building trust and SEO juice and 2) start a keep-in-touch plan to fertilize your seeds, you'll have completed the first crucial steps towards set-it-and-forget-it marketing and being a gardener rather than a scavenger.

Chapter 11

Patient Rapport and Retention

Let's talk more about patient rapport and retention. This is a crucial and foundational piece to a successful practice that will allow you to avoid the never-ending hamster wheel of constant marketing. It lets the world know that we mean business.

In order to feel secure and stable in your practice, and to avoid the drastic, cyclical swings that make you feel worried about what next week will look like, you need to have a high degree of patient retention. You want to keep them around. You don't want your office to be a revolving door of patients coming and constantly going out. You want them to come in, join the party, and stay for as long as it takes to help them get better.

I'm not talking about being salesy, or trying to push big packages on people. No, I'm talking about educating and priming them to do what's in their best interest. You owe it to your patients to make it easy for them to stick around long enough to experience the ultimate benefits of your care. We know that acupuncture is a cumulative medicine that can take 6-12 treatments to produce results. We also know that prevention is the best medicine, and that our medicine can help so many people to feel better and improve their lives, but they need to get in regularly to gain its benefits.

Patient retention comes down to how you're educating your patients about acupuncture, building their expectations and trust, and on-boarding them so they commit to the full course of treatment that's best for them.

Here is a simple and easy hack for gently and consistently reminding your patients of your value (and the desirability of your services) every single time they come to see you. When you're inserting needles, tell them in a nutshell what each point is for, and make sure you're linking it to their symptoms, complaints, and goals (i.e., their values). For example, "This point, although it's in your ankle, is actually for your shoulder pain! This point is to help with stress and to support your liver, and this point is for your digestion." They don't need to know that Spleen 6 is called *Three Yin Intersection*, and they don't need to know all that it can do; they just need to know why I've chosen it for them specifically.

This reminds them that you are working on their problems and goals, and it also involves them in their care, which is important to me. It bothers me that so much of a patient's power is taken away in Western medicine. I want to empower and educate and inspire my patients. And I also want to remind them of what I'm doing, plus a little bit of *why* and *how*. They should walk out feeling like they know what just went down.

Suppose you referred a friend to an acupuncturist, only to learn that acupuncturist wasn't an effective communicator. Your friend leaves the office unsure of what the acupuncturist did or what the plan is. Ohmylordy, that's so disappointing and disempowering, and I doubt that friend would return for a follow-up treatment. This is because your friend wasn't made to understand clearly how the treatment was linked to their values, problems, and goals. The acupuncturist expected them to just blindly trust the vague, confusing, and foreign process that they don't understand (kind of like Western medicine does, but without the benefit of the implicit respect and trust that doctors have simply by being a doctor). So, that's a simple and easy hack for gently reminding patients of the value and benefits of your care – tell them what's going on in a way they understand.

In acupuncture, the transition from skeptical prospect to committed patient typically happens within the first two visits. During that time, people are doing their best to decide whether or not they're in the right place. In this section, I'm going to guide you through the psychology of the intake process.

The better you are at connecting with your patients and finding out exactly why they've come to you, the more successful you'll be at securing their commitment to the full course of treatment.

The famous Paredo Principle, also known as the 80/20 rule, states that 80% of the results in virtually any system come from 20% of the activity. In the scenario of our clinics, this means that what happens in the first 20% of a person's interaction with us and our office will most likely influence 80% of their future experience with us! Your intake process is priming them for their future experience with you. It's shaping their expectations. If your intake process is warm, organized, clear, specific, efficient, personal and professional, then your client is preparing for a future relationship based on that experience. If your intake is just the quick and dirty, they'll prepare for a future experience of "quick and dirty". If it feels like you are uncomfortable or insecure, they'll prepare for a future experience of the same.

When it comes to your patient's decision-making process, how you gather and present information in your intake process becomes almost more important than the information itself. You can build rapport, connection, and understanding along the way with your questioning. You're educating them about the way we look at symptoms in the body, and the way everything is related and connected through the questions you ask. The way you analyze and clarify what they tell you indicates to them that you are a detective, and that you're on their team. The way you listen to them in an approachable, confident and compassionate manner, never judging, preaching or coming off as arrogant, will influence the degree to which they will trust you.

This is all to say that the intake process is critically important for educating your patients and priming them to stick around and commit to treatment. Next, I'll tell you about the 5-step initial intake template, so you can master this process.

The "It's all about them" 6-step initial intake template

When people show up to your practice, they're coming because they want their health problems to be different, better, improved or enhanced in some way. They are experiencing a challenge or concern of some kind, and although they might find you interesting, inspiring, captivating or uplifting, they're not in your office for you. They are in your office because they want a result, an outcome, or a benefit for themselves. Therefore, your initial client intake and consultation needs to be *all about them*, because that's what they care about.

The following template is a very effective format for quickly establishing rapport and getting to the real reason that they are seeking your help at this time.

There are five stages to the intake. Be sure to follow them in order. Each stage involves asking questions.

"Pretend that every single
person you meet has a
sign around his or her neck that
says, 'Make me feel
important,'... and you will
succeed in life."

— Mary Kay Ash

Step 1. Connect with them and establish rapport.

Establish rapport by acknowledging them, welcoming them and thanking them for coming.

- Greet or introduce yourself. Hi! My name is Katie, what's your name? Make sure you introduce yourself with a SMILE. People form opinions within the first three to five seconds of meeting you, so your voice, your eye contact, and manner are crucial here. Similarities forge bonds. The quicker you can ask people questions about their lives that lead to common threads between you and them, the easier it is to build rapport.

Step 2: Identify their need.

Ask them what *they* think the problem is

- What's their primary or immediate need? Find out what appears to be missing or problematic in their lives. The better you are doing this, the more committed they will be to your practice.

- Ask them what brought them in, what they think is going on, and what they are concerned or worried about. You want to find out their truly compelling reason for coming to you, not just what they may have listed as their chief complaint on their forms. What is their real motivator? What do they really want a solution to?

Step 3: Confirm their need.

Be certain you've established their true need. Repeat it back to them. Don't assume or guess.

Step 4: Ask them what *they* think the solution should be.

- What do they think needs to happen? Listen.

- What is their opinion about what's really going on? What do they think is the "cause" or the contributing factors?

- Ask them what process they think they should be going through. What steps do they think they'll need to go through in order to get where they want to go?

- This is a coaching technique that, by getting the client involved in their own solution, makes them more motivated and likely to commit to taking action for themselves. It's an important psychology.

Step 5: Ask all of your normal questions to formulate your differential diagnosis and treatment plan.

Explain to them that you're going to ask them a bunch of questions, and while they may seem unrelated to their chief complaint, they're relevant to you, and you need to get a solid understanding of the patient, their constitution and their pattern so that you can get to the root of the problem.

Step 6: Offer value and make your recommendation.

This is when you get to let your TCM genius fly. Give them your report of findings and your solution. Explain your diagnosis in a language they can understand. People generally love to learn about themselves. This is where you can really wow them if you do it right. Most people struggle with their issues for a while before coming to us. Usually, they haven't received a good explanation that makes sense. No one's told them that they don't have a bunch of different diseases or problems, but just one underlying pattern that is related to all the different symptoms, and that to you their complex array of seemingly separate symptoms all make perfect sense. They don't have dry eyes, insomnia, night sweats, fatigue, AND restless leg syndrome, for example, they are just a little yin and blood deficient. Once we address that, ALL of their symptoms should improve! If you can explain this to them in a language and manner they are able to understand, this will blow them away. You will be the answer to their prayers.

This is also when you give them your recommendation. Let them know that you think acupuncture can help them. Estimate how many treatments you think it will take and how frequently they need to come. Say it clearly, directly, and confidently.

Through all of this, you are "onboarding" them into your process, all while educating them about themselves! It inspires them, gives them hope, and builds their trust in you.

And then you get them on the table, and they are so excited for your treatment!

Remember, through this whole intake process, your patients are thinking:

- Do I really believe she understands my problem and can deliver a solution?
- Do I feel safe with her? Do I like and trust her?
- Do I believe she can help me get results I desire, and is she worth the cost?

Tailor your work as a solution to their issue. If someone says they can't afford something, that only means that you haven't demonstrated value in their terms, so communicate more value. What I mean by that is, say they come to you with a problem, and while you asked them a million questions, you never really seemed to hone in on or reiterate that you understand their chief complaint. And even worse, you instead talked a ton about their gut, their spleen, and their bowel movements. Even though this is relevant to their chief complaint, if you have not showed them that you understand their chief complaint, linking their gut (in this example) to it, they will feel completely unheard. And when you make your recommendation to come back eight times to fix their gut, they won't see the value in it. This approach does not speak to them in terms of their values. They'll say they can't afford it.

In order to show your patient that the treatment is valuable, you must directly and explicitly link it to their problem and desired outcome, not something vague or completely irrelevant to their primary complaint.

This requires the ability to listen, so listen carefully and humbly, and tailor your questions to fit your patients' responses and needs. Link your services to your patients' specific needs, values, and desires, and your services will sell themselves. Be sincere and genuinely interested. Keep the focus on them.

It's all about building relationships with your potential clients on the basis of trust. It's about having a sincere conversation that allows you to let your patients know what you can do to help them. It all starts with a simple conversation in which you are listening to detect their need and if you can help them, and they are listening to see if you can help provide a solution to their need, and the appropriate amount of trust and understanding is assured.

The 5 most common mistakes acupuncturists make when delivering their ROF... and how to avoid them

1. The biggest mistake practitioners make when delivering their report of findings is that they don't have a practiced system and method for how they talk about and educate patients about acupuncture, how it works, what to expect, etc.

    Solution: Prepare, prepare, prepare! Preparation is the "mother of success". Create a ROF script and drill it on a regular basis until you own it! It should be short, concise, simple, and delivered confidently.

2. They don't really listen to their patient. Instead, they focus on things that are important to them, but not necessarily important to their client.

    Solution: Be consultative. Lead your patient with your questions, and then listen to what they are telling you.

3. They don't clearly define the problem that they are solving in terms that are obvious and meaningful to the client.

    Solution: Explain to the patient what the diagnosis is, in a way that the patient can understand.

In some cases, you don't need to tell them a TCM diagnosis. For pain especially, you can usually just say, "Acupuncture is great at treating back pain. I think we can help" or "I think inflammation and poor circulation are driving your pain, and acupuncture is great at reducing inflammation and increasing circulation, so that's what we're going to do". But sometimes, I think it's helpful to give them a quick and dirty TCM diagnosis, such as: "Here's what I think is going on: Your migraines are being caused by too little yin anchoring the yang, so we need to anchor your yang and nourish yin." Use analogies to help them understand what you mean. I usually say something like, "I know, our language in Chinese medicine is so weird." What they need to see is that you have an understanding, a process, and a plan. You're not just randomly throwing needles and taking their money. And you're not focusing on treating something they don't care about; you're focusing on fixing their big, pressing problem. We may think that should be obvious to our patients, but it's not.

4. They don't clearly articulate their vision of HOW they are going to deliver the solution. They don't tell them, "This is what it will be like. This is exactly what you can expect. We'll do this, then you'll feel this, then…"

   Solution: When you make recommendations for care, break it down for your patients. Explain the process and why you propose to do things the way you do. Let them know that the reason is to give them the best result possible. Then, give them a play-by-play of what they can expect and in what time frame. This is known as "future-pacing." You're creating a tangible and compelling future for them, first in their mind, then laying out a *way* to get there.

   I tell them that if their problem has been going on a while, it will take more time to unravel it, and that I need to see them regularly. I explain that we don't want to take a step forward with each treatment and then take a step back in the long gap between appointments. We want to make progress, so I need to see them regularly with appointments not too far apart. I draw them a little graph of how symptoms usually resolve. I say it can take a few treatments until we've reached the right cumulative dosage for them to notice any improvement, and they might only notice small improvements in relaxation and sleep in the meantime. And then, once we hit the tipping point and they do start seeing improvement, if they notice symptoms returning, then we've gone too long between treatments. People usually understand this. It makes perfect sense, and I don't feel like I'm being a salesy person who's trying to sell them on more than they need. They can feel I have their best interest at heart, and understand the process and what to expect. They can feel my hope and optimism for them. This gets them excited and inspired to commit to the treatment plan.

5. They focus on the features of their technique and how they do what they do, but they don't paint a vivid picture of the benefits of those features: what their patients will get, experience or be able to do because of the care.

    Solution: Paint a very specific picture of what their life will be like if and when they follow your recommendations.

    What do you expect them to experience or feel after working with you? What will they feel when they first start working with you? What would they notice changing? How will they feel after a few weeks, or after a few months? What will they be experiencing by the time they got to the end of your plan for them? How often will they need to see you? What will they need to do or avoid doing to get the best possible results?

The answer to confusion
is always no.

When you have clearly articulated these benefits, your ROF will be irresistible.

If your office systems and communication are top-notch, and if you've compassionately listened to and shown that you understand and care about solving their problem, then you have just about sealed the deal by the time your patients get to the report of findings.

Many practitioners avoid telling their patients the truth about what they think is in the patient's best interest because they don't want to deal with rejection, or they're afraid of sounding bossy, or they're afraid of being wrong. The truth is, when what you want is the best result possible for your patients – and you own your value and feel totally congruent and excited about what you offer—you won't even have to think about how to respond to rejection; your patients are paying you to guide them and give them a plan. That's exactly what they want from you; it's not being "bossy".

If you think you don't have enough experience, or that this person won't follow-through, or they'll think you charge too much, or if you don't think you're worth it, then why should they? You've got to believe in yourself and this medicine, because they're both amazing.

Thinking of yourself as an authority

For new grads, one of the hardest parts of starting an acupuncture practice is stepping into an authoritative role. You are used to having your clinic supervisor there to lean on and look to. Many of you even had clinic partners whom you co-treated with. Now, you are on your own. You are in control, and you are the authority. So, let me remind you: You know your medicine, you know what is best for your patients in terms of your medicine, and it is your job to educate them.

"Other people tend to value you the way you value yourself."

— Lee Miller

This is one of the biggest mistakes I see acupuncturists make. They are too loosey-goosey with their patients, letting them take the reins in terms of their care. I know, I get it, I too had to learn it the hard way. I remember when I first started out, I would say to my patient, "So, when do you want to come back?" And I had several patients say to me, "I don't know, what do you think – you're the doctor!" And I was like, "Oh yeah! I'm the expert here!" Don't make that same mistake I did. Proactively step into your role as the authority before your patients have to remind you.

Jay Abrahams, a business executive and author, has a philosophy he calls The Strategy of Preeminence, which I'll briefly paraphrase:

- It is your job as a business owner and practitioner to lead, advise, and serve your clients in those clients' best interests.

- It is your responsibility to tell it as you see it. (In other words, don't hold back in telling them what you know from your experience, which will get them the best results.)

- Never let someone just do whatever they want when it comes to using your services if it is not in their best interest.

- Your goal is to become a trusted advisor. Don't allow patients to settle for a visit frequency that won't produce the results they need.

- You're doing your clients a disservice if you don't impart your wisdom to them and share what you know can help them.

- Be dedicated to having an impact on your clients' lives. Provide solutions to problems or challenges they feel emotionally as well as rationally.

- Acknowledge, respect and communicate the value of what you have done, are doing and will do for your clients down the road, so that they can understand the significance of what it means in their lives.

If you want to be known as an expert, then it is critical that you proactively communicate your wisdom and your value to your patients in a language that they can relate to. You are the expert! I cannot stress this enough. Most acupuncturists make the mistake of assuming that people have a pretty good idea of what they offer and how it works, but being a pro means leaving nothing to assumption.

If you're letting your patients do whatever they wish in terms of your care, then you are doing them a huge disservice. Because *they* are not the expert, *you* are.

It's your responsibility to advise your patients in their best interest. As an expert.

An expert who can make a very personalized recommendation for them, taking into account their goals, their history, your knowledge of your medicine and your experience.

Do you know that that's what everyone wants - to be personally advised by a confident and compassionate expert? Even if your patients don't realize that's what they want, they need and deserve a personalized recommendation from an expert that will help them get the results they want. It's your responsibility to give it to them.

As an acupuncturist, you must dose your medicine. You must make recommendations as to when your patient needs to come back and how frequently they should be getting treatments, and you must give them an estimate of how many treatments they should expect it to take.

This is practicing good medicine. It's just as much your job as inserting needles.

If you're not doing this, it would be like a doctor giving their patient antibiotics and not telling them how many to take or when to take them. It's reckless, and it's not best for the patient.

How many acupuncture treatments will it take?

It can be difficult, if not downright impossible, to predict exactly the moment when your patient will experience significant improvement in their symptoms. The good news is that you don't need to predict it precisely; you're not a magician or fortune teller and that's not what they're expecting from you. But you do need to give an estimation.

The following guidelines will help estimate the number of required treatments:

1. How long have the symptoms been going on? The longer they've been around, the more treatments it will take.

2. How old is the patient? The older they are, the more treatments it will take.

3. Are symptoms consistent? If symptoms are constant, for example, a constant 4/10 on the pain scale, the more treatments it will take. If symptoms are variable, for example, sometimes a 2/10 and sometimes 8/10, it will take fewer treatments.

4. How is the patient progressing? You can continue to tweak your estimation as you work with the patient and update your expectations and recommendations based on what you see. There is a beginning, middle, and end to a course of treatment. The beginning is how many treatments it takes for them to start seeing improvement. The middle is where you make most of the progress. And the end is making it stick. If the beginning stage takes longer, you know the middle stage will take longer, too. You can adjust expectations based on this progress you see.

When in doubt, I recommend telling patients that it should take around 6-8 treatments.

This gives you enough time to at least make *some* improvements. By 6-8 treatments, most patients are at least seeing some improvement, if not a significant improvement, in some or all of their symptoms. And this is all they need to make them want to stick around, even if you haven't yet completely solved all of their problems. (For fertility, specifically, I tell patients to expect about 3-4 months of treatment).

You've got to confidently and compassionately insist, guide, and lead them to receive the number and frequency of treatments that are appropriate for them; the number that will help them get the results they desire.

Don't do what I did in my first few months of practice and fail to give patients a recommendation or plan. If they'd insist that I give them my recommendation, I'd hesitantly say, "Let's give it 3 treatments and see how you do." Forehead smack! Three was often not enough! I feel badly that I led those patients poorly, and that they might have left my office after three treatments thinking acupuncture couldn't help them. I really did them a disservice.

It's because I lacked confidence and training in how to effectively dose my medicine.

I don't want you to make the same mistakes I did. Please have confidence in yourself and our amazing medicine, and dose your medicine appropriately to advise your patients in their best interest.

To help you do this, I surveyed 200 acupuncturists about their experiences in terms of how many sessions it usually takes to see significant and lasting improvement for various symptoms. What I found is that, on average, it takes about 8-10 treatments to see results. If you'd like to know more, you can see the results of that survey here:

https://acuprosper.com/acupuncture-dosage/

Please don't underestimate yourself, and please don't underestimate your medicine. Our medicine is amazing. When given in a therapeutic dosage, it really can perform what seem like miracles. Don't shortchange yourself, your medicine, or your patient by failing to recommend the appropriate number of treatments to get results. Patients need you to guide them in this. They won't come back frequently enough unless you tell them to.

At many acupuncture schools, students are limited to working on a patient in clinic for a maximum of six treatments. The thinking behind it is that they want students to gain a variety of experience in treating patients. However, when you look at the data stating that it takes on average 8-10 treatments to make a significant improvement in a condition, it's not surprising that many students are finding themselves doubting their own abilities or their medicine. They haven't been given the chance to see the dramatic results their treatments can make on peoples' health and lives. That's so sad. So please, listen to me when I tell you that you are a great practitioner, and this medicine is powerful. Give it a chance. And to give it a chance, you must learn to confidently recommend an adequate number of treatments for your patients.

So, remember: You are an authority. Advise your patients based on your expertise. They want and need you to do that. If you don't feel like an authority, then take some continuing education classes, read books, get your hands on more people, and make sure you have the confidence and expertise you need. This isn't about faking it until you make it, but I want to remind you that you've had extensive schooling and practice, and you know a TON more than you realize. One of the beautiful things about our medicine is that there is SO much to learn. We will never be bored and know it all, and that excites me, but don't let that undermine how much you ALREADY know. Especially compared to your patients, who know NOTHING about this medicine. YOU are in charge!

While it may feel uncomfortable at first, you've got to get comfortable saying, "I think I can help, and here's what I recommend".

This is not bragging; this is what your patients NEED to hear from you. Bragging is about comparing yourself to others and proclaiming your superiority. Declaring your strengths, your skills, your expertise, and your ability to help is not bragging, but expressing confidence in what your potential clients expect, want, and need to hear from you.

If the thought of establishing yourself as an expert immediately induces a sense of panic, you're not alone. For many of us, this can trigger our self-doubt and insecurities. You'll know your inner critic has taken over when thoughts start frantically racing around inside your head like, "Who am I to call myself an expert? What do I know? I don't know enough yet." Does this sound familiar? I'll bet it does, and you're not alone in this experience.

It's called the "imposter syndrome" – the phenomenon of highly capable people being plagued by self-doubt. It's incredibly common for both men and women, but I think it's more extreme for women. Tina Fey has admitted to these feelings. So have Meryl Streep, Kate Winslet, Maya Angelou, and the list goes on. I think as humans, and especially as women, we all consistently underestimate ourselves.

So, if you're feeling this, please know that you're not alone. Everyone experiences it. But please don't listen to this inner critic inside your head. Don't try to silence it, because unfortunately, it will probably never be silenced. Every time you challenge yourself to grow, dare yourself to try something new or go for a dream, your inner critic will very likely rear her very mean head. We can't silence her. We can only move on in spite of her, lovingly bringing her along for the ride with us. Liz Gilbert wrote about this beautifully in her book *Big Magic*. I highly recommend it if you'd like to read more about getting past your inner critic.

It takes vulnerability to step up with courage in the face of uncertainty. By having confidence, I don't mean you've got to say, "100% all your problems will be solved, I'm God's gift, I'm amazing." No, that's arrogance, not confidence. Confidence is, even in the face of self-doubt, saying, "I've never treated this before, but I think we can help, and here's what it's going to take, and here's what my plan is for helping you." Do you see the difference? You don't have to be arrogant. You can still be honest, saying, "I don't know, but here's what I think it's going to take". With leadership, expertise, and effectively dosing your medicine, you can still deliver results with an earnest and humble approach.

Over time, I learned to trust and have confidence in myself and my medicine. Largely, I learned this from my patients who courageously and stubbornly insisted on coming back, even when I failed to lead them. Through seeing them and the results they got, I learned, "Whoa, okay, I can do this, and wow, my medicine really does work. This is awesome." And I slowly learned to have confidence.

I believe that you've got to believe in yourself and work on cultivating your confidence. But I think that saying, "Oh, you've got to believe in yourself," isn't totally accurate, and it actually can be disempowering, because it doesn't necessarily leave room for uncertainty. I want you to know that self-doubt and uncertainty are just, for most of us, part of the process and the journey. And I see so many acupuncturists say things like, "Well, first I've got to just work on myself and visualize getting clarity and confidence before I can even start to learn how to market my practice."

I don't think that sitting and thinking is the answer to this uncertainty and self-doubt. The antidote to these is getting your hands on people and stepping into action. That is how you learn to believe in yourself - getting your hands on people and seeing, "Oh my gosh, our medicine actually works."

There's a difference between saying, "I've got all the answers," and saying, "I'm not sure, but I think we can help, and here's what it's going to take." And the difference is courage - Brené Brown style courage. It takes vulnerability to, in the face of an uncertain outcome, still really show up. It takes vulnerability and courage to bravely risk failure. And with time, it gets easier. As you see your medicine work again and again, it gets easier to say, "I'm not sure, but I think we can help. Never treated this before, but I think we can help, and here's what it's going to take."

It's just like with flight attendants on an airplane. If they're freaked out by the turbulence, everyone on the plane is going to be super freaked out. They're the leaders. If they're calm, everyone else feels calmer. As the acupuncturist, leader and expert, if you don't have hope and you say, "I don't know, might not work, let's give it one try and see." Then at no point is your patient going to have hope, show up, and reschedule.

But even if you say, "I don't know, but I think we can help and here's my plan," and think to yourself, I'm willing to risk failure and have courage because I have hope in my patient's healing and I think they deserve a fair shot, they are going to feel that. They'll be more likely to say, "Okay, let's do it." You are the leader, so it's crucial that you build trust with people.

The more people you treat, the more you'll be blown away by our medicine, and you'll see that you - little, imperfect you and me, with so much more to learn - can effectively harness the power of this incredible medicine. So, I want you to believe in yourself.

I also, though, want you to know that if you have self-doubt and uncertainty, you are not alone, and you are absolutely okay. I want you to have courage in the face of that self-doubt and uncertainty.

If some other side of you is whining, "Do I have to? Do I have to think of myself as an expert?" the answer is a firm and resounding, "Yes, you do!" Like it or not, becoming an expert isn't optional if you want your practice to be as successful as it can be. It's a must. Becoming an expert will create the trust necessary for potential patients to feel comfortable and confident about working with you and following your advice.

I think it's helpful to choose an area or two to really dig into and become an expert in. Even if your clinic doesn't have a specialty or niche, you can still hone your skills and specialize in a few conditions that you love to treat. Identify and focus on a condition or two that you want to be known for, and that you want to treat more of.

Exercise: Please answer the following questions.

1. In what areas are you currently an expert? What conditions have you gotten awesome results for? What conditions do you love to treat?

   _____

   _____

2. If there were ONE thing you could be known for treating, what would it be?

   _____

   _____

3. What do you need to LEARN to feel more confident in the area you'd like to be known for?

_____

_____

4. List the ways in which you could learn these things – CEUs, books, training programs, apprenticing a mentor, etc.

_____

_____

Even if you're already very knowledgeable about your specialty, continue to learn and stay up to date with the latest information. Read at least one book a month on your chosen subject, which will increase your knowledge, challenge you to see a different perspective, or spark new ideas and thoughts, all of which will enhance the value you provide your patients.

You must make the crucial mental shift of thinking of yourself as an expert. If YOU don't believe it, you'll have a hard time persuading anyone else to believe it. Begin to think of and refer to yourself as an expert in your chosen specialty. Begin to view your role with your patients as that of a highly important and trusted advisor.

Confidence and uncertainty

There are a lot of limiting beliefs that can hold us back. Self-doubt, what other people think, the "supposed-tos," the "shoulds," and the desire for perfection. This will inevitably lead to anxiety, disempowered thinking, and fear. I talk a lot about self-doubt because that's what I personally have dealt with it, and I still deal with it all the time.

But here's another self-limiting belief that will surprise you. It surprised me too when I started to notice it with the acupuncturists that I teach. What is it? It's the discomfort of uncertainty.

I see this pop up in two ways in our acupuncture clinics. Will my treatments work? Will I be able to help this patient? What if it doesn't work? I care about this person, and I don't want to waste their time or their money; what if I can't help them? We acupuncturists are caring people with such good intentions, and that can lead to so much self-imposed pressure. That self-doubt leads to the fear, "What if I can't help them?"

These personal uncertainties lead to professional uncertainties: What if my clinic doesn't grow? What if I build it and no one comes? What if I'm not good at this? Will my business work? Will I be able to support myself? Will everyone think I'm a failure if it doesn't work?

These uncertainties are scary. It's incredibly uncomfortable. Both of these (will my treatment be successful and will my business be successful) cannot be guaranteed. And the discomfort of the uncertainty can cause us to self-sabotage, or to look for ways to escape from that uncertainty, and therefore to not really go for it or give it a fair shot. How does this manifest? In not confidently investing in what it takes to succeed – not telling your patients that you think you can help. Not describing to them how many treatments you think it will take or how frequently they need to come back to really give it a fair shot and an effective dosage.

Because even the most skilled acupuncturist can't know for certain exactly how many treatments it will take, proposing a treatment to patients can feel really uncomfortable. I felt this when I first started, and I see this in the acupuncturist whom I employ and coach: that fear of being wrong driven by that uncertainty.

you've got to be willing
to show up in ways that
make you uncomfortable

But that's how healing is. It's uncertain. It's the same with medicine, drugs, and surgery. It's the same with therapy. It's the same with love. It's the same with life. There's inherent uncertainty, and it's uncomfortable.

When I was in graduate school, I worked as a rafting guide on the weekends. I loved being on the river ever since I read Siddhartha in high school, but it was a really scary job. I was guiding families through class-four whitewater rapids; despite my prowess, the water was unpredictable. One bump, and they could fall out of the boat, hit their heads on a rock and drown. So, it was a lot of responsibility and uncertainty, right? The river is powerful, and it's changing all the time.

At the same time, I was also working as an office manager for a homeopath and chiropractor. One time, she and her family came rafting with me one day, and she said something to me that I've never forgotten. She said, "This job is really going to help you be a better acupuncturist."

I met those words with a blank stare. I didn't understand the connection between raft guiding and being an acupuncturist. She clarified, "Your ability to courageously lead people through such uncertainty is going to help you to be a better practitioner." Years later, once I graduated and went into practice for myself, I understood what she meant.

There's uncertainty in our job as healers. We have to courageously lead people through that uncertainty. It's our job to be their leaders. Just as I was yelling "forward paddle" as a rafting guide to my crew, we are saying, "We can help. Let's get you rescheduled next week." We are saying "onward" too, to our patients.

So, what's the way out of this discomfort? It's actually to lean into that uncertainty. To hold space for it. Sit with it. Allow it. It's okay. Remember that with holistic medicine, it's about the patients healing themselves. We're choosing where the needles go. We're facilitating it, but their bodies are healing themselves. Take some pressure off of yourself.

In order to give your patients an actual fighting chance of getting results, you must guide them to coming back frequently enough to get those results.

If you have an energy of doubt and fear, it will play into your patients' fears too. If you don't display confidence in your medicine, they most certainly will not either. They won't schedule a follow-up treatment with you after their first visit, or they just won't show up for their scheduled visits. You've got to be a beacon of hope.

Get comfortable with that discomfort of uncertainty, and learn to courageously exude confidence in the face of it. That's what it takes for your patients to succeed. You've got to tell them, "Yes, I can help, and here's what it'll take. Here's my plan." You've got to dose your medicine enough to get those results.

Imagine if you went to a doctor for, say, a broken ankle, and your doctor said, "Keep the cast on for two days…two months…I don't know, whatever you think." Just like with acupuncture, the doctor can't know exactly the moment when your bone will be healed so that you can take the cast off. But if they don't give you a definitive and conservative framework, then they're not doing their job, and you would not have faith in their recommendation - you wouldn't know what action to take. You would be very unlikely to keep that cast on long enough to heal and get the results you need.

If they underestimate, instead of overestimating the time they think it would take you to heal, they would also be making a grave mistake, potentially costing you that healing opportunity. And it's the same with us in our acupuncture treatments. Wouldn't you rather be the person who says, "I believe you can do this" and potentially be wrong, than be the person who says, "I don't think we can do this" and be right?

The best and most successful acupuncturists are the ones who have become comfortable with that uncertainty. Even though they've been in business for many, many years, and have seen many, many people get better, they still don't know *for certain* that they're going to help that person. They still don't know for certain how many treatments it's going to take. They've gotten comfortable with that not knowing. They've gotten comfortable with some discomfort.

In order to rise up and do great things, you've got to get comfortable with discomfort. You've got to be willing to be uncomfortable.

Let go of the ego's fear of being wrong. Get comfortable with that uncertainty. Courage is a muscle. Practice it and grow it. It gets easier. The longer you're in practice, the more you see your medicine working to improve your patients. It gets easier to confidently say, "Yes, I think I can help, and here's how many treatments I'm expecting it to take." It does get easier to say, "I'm not discouraged. This is what I'd expect," when a patient checks in with you after not seeing improvement on their second or third treatment. If, in that scenario, you don't lead with confidence and hope, and you're discouraged, uncertain, and worried that you might be wrong, then they're out of there. That patient will not stick around long enough to get the results that you could get them if you had confidently led them.

You've got to get comfortable with the uncertainty and tell them that yes, you can help, even when it's not guaranteed. It's uncertain. Now, of course, refer out if you really don't think you can help. You have a responsibility to refer out in this case, but you can really help and do amazing things with your medicine. So please, don't underestimate yourself or your medicine.

Putting yourself out there and taking risks actually builds confidence and strength. The more you do it, the more confident you will become. You can't gain confidence any other way.

It's courage and fear,
not courage or fear.

Chapter 12

The Little Voice Inside your Head...

"What you believe about yourself
and your life, on a deep subconscious
level is what you live out daily
through your actions, words, choices,
and habits. It's also what you attract
and manifest more of. Be mindful
of the power of your beliefs and
their power over your life."

— Lala Delia

We've talked about stepping into your authority and confidence, imposter syndrome, and getting comfortable with the discomfort of uncertainty. The little voice inside our heads deserves even more discussion, however, because it's so powerful.

I want to tell you about a secret superpower you have: Your distinctly human ability to make stuff up and believe in stories that are not necessarily true. According to the author of a book called *Sapiens: A Brief History of Humankind*, this ability to create and believe in stories is unique to humans, and one of the traits that has led to our dominance on the planet. We have collective stories and beliefs that we all agree to believe in – things like nations, money, and laws – that create a framework for our lives.

We also use stories on a personal level. Each of us is living by stories and beliefs that are unique to us and similarly creating a framework for our lives - even if these stories and beliefs are subconscious (which they often are). Here's an example: We might tell ourselves that most people are dishonest, even though that's not an absolute fact. Obviously, not everyone is dishonest. If that's a belief you have, then that will become the world you live in. Because that will be what your brain chooses to focus on and act on.

Stories and beliefs are your mental map of the world. They are the lens through which you experience and interpret the world around you. They are the filter through which you perceive your reality. The quality of your stories determines the quality of your life.

I'm sure you've heard of the placebo effect. It's often used as a way to discount the effectiveness of certain medical treatments, but I see it as proof of just how powerful beliefs are.

What is the placebo effect? In medicine, it's simply a beneficial effect produced by a substance or treatment that has no known curative properties, and is therefore due to the patient's belief in the treatment, not the treatment itself. The placebo effect proves scientifically, beyond a shadow of a doubt, that our beliefs actually change our physical reality.

Beliefs even have the power to override the effects of drugs. An experiment by Dr. Henry Beecher of Harvard University showed that when people were given a stimulating drug but told it was a sedative (or vice versa), half of the participants experienced symptoms that matched their *expectations* of the drug, not the drug itself. These weren't placebo pills the participants were given - they were actual drugs. That demonstrates how powerful our minds are.

The point here is that beliefs are powerful. Your beliefs affect so many different aspects of your life, it's incredible. Some of the main ones are your emotions, your behavior, how you respond to situations, what you focus on, your perspective, and the meaning you give to things that happen. All these are affected by your beliefs.

Let's say, for example, that you have a limiting belief that says, "There's nothing I can do to change my situation." You'd have no optimism, and it's likely that opportunities may not be visible to you. You would focus on what you lack - how bad your situation is. What kind of meaning would you attach to the events in your life? They would be proof to you that you can't change anything. You'd see things as signs that you can't move forward.

Now, let's turn the tables. Suppose you had the empowering belief that said, "I create my own reality." You'd probably act more often. You'd get off the couch and go. You'd do stuff excitedly and enthusiastically. You'd probably act confidently, because you would know you have the power to change things. You'd have a sense of control, optimism, and excitement, because you would that know you have the power to shape your world. You'd probably respond to situations creatively, resourcefully, and positively. You'd be better able to recognize opportunities around you because you're in a more positive and creative energy state. You'd focus on what you already have: your progress, your goals, self-improvement, and the good things going on in your life. You'd think that whatever happened to you is more proof that you create your own reality. So, you see how our stories can affect so many different aspects of our life.

The difference between empowering stories and limiting stories is that empowering stories allow us to move forward in our lives and do what we want to do; limiting stories, on the other hand, hold us back.

What stories are you telling yourself?

The first step to taking control of what's going on inside our heads is to uncover exactly what's really going on in there.

Typically, when people are being productive, feeling inspired, and making progress, the thoughts inside our heads are positive. And typically, when people are unproductive and overwhelmed, their thoughts tend to be harsh and negative: "It's too much", "It's not worth the effort", or "I'm not good enough." The thing is, we all think and feel these things from time to time, and that's normal and fine. The problem arises when we get stuck there – when we don't check in with ourselves. This allows these thoughts to determine the decisions we make and actions we take.

When I'm asking myself to expand, but I feel stuck, frustrated, and in a funk, I use the following exercise to uncover what could be keeping me stuck.

"I AM," two of the most powerful words. For what you put after them shapes your reality."

— Bevan Lee

The first step to changing your limiting beliefs is to first find out what they are! Uncovering your limiting stories is so powerful that, sometimes, it's the only step needed to eliminate them.

1. Choose one or more areas of your life where you feel stuck, meaning you're not getting the results you want. (Perhaps it's career, finances, family, health, romance, social, spiritual, personal growth, education, and so on.)

   _____

   _____

   Here are some common frustrations, just to get your creative juices flowing:

   "I'm stuck, in a rut"; "I have no life. I'm burned out – exhausted"; "I'm frustrated and discouraged"; "I'm just not making enough to make ends meet. I never seem to get ahead"; "Maybe I just don't have what it takes"; "I'm not making a difference"; "I feel empty inside. My life lacks meaning; something's missing"; "I'm stressed out. Everything's urgent"; "I can't change things".

2. In a single sentence, identify and describe the specific problem you're having in each area. (Examples: I'm not making enough money; I don't feel confident; I feel isolated and alone.)

   _____

   _____

3. Look at your above sentence and add the word "because" to the end. Then, complete each sentence out loud as quickly as possible, and don't judge the answer. What you say after the word "because" will give you a clue as to

what your underlying, limiting beliefs are. Write your statements here:

_____

_____

4. Repeat this process several times for each statement - it's likely you will have several limiting beliefs or stories around the same issue.

_____

_____

Here's a personal example: I was asked to give a graduation speech for acupuncturists at CSTCM. The day before I gave the talk, I realized I was getting nervous. I decided to do this exercise to find out what beliefs were causing this emotion. These were what I uncovered:

"I'm nervous for my talk because I'm afraid I might not give valuable or inspiring enough information." Clearly, at the root of that is a story I'm telling myself that reads, "I'm not enough. I'm not good enough". Simply recognizing this belief allowed me to coach and visualize myself past that belief.

As a side note, you can uncover your empowering stories by doing the same above exercises, but in step 1, choosing areas of your life where you feel things are going well, or that you're already successful in. And then, continue with the rest of the steps in the exercise. You will see the positive stories about yourself in the process, so way to go on those! But let's continue focusing on honing in on and shifting the negative beliefs.

The question you need to always be asking yourself is this: Are my stories empowering me, or are they holding me back? We can change our beliefs. It's our responsibility to choose beliefs that empower us.

The next step, honing in on your limiting belief, requires you to ask yourself, "Why does this seem true to me?". Pretend that no one but you is responsible for any problem you have. This doesn't mean that your problems are your *fault*, but that they are your *responsibility*.

5. Take the statements you wrote down in step 4 above and answer each "why" until you can no longer come up with any more reasonable responses.

   Example: "I'm nervous because I believe I'm not good enough."

   Why does this seem true? Because my parents never paid attention to me.

   Because I've delivered a terrible speech in the past.

   As an alternative to "Why does this seem true?" you could also ask: "Why is this an issue for me"; "Why does this bother me"; "Why do I think this is a problem"; and "Why do I feel like that?"

   _____

   _____

Next, in order to begin dismantling this limiting belief, you want to find evidence to the contrary. Tony Robbins, in his book *Awaken the Giant Within*, gives the analogy of beliefs being like tables. I prefer to think of beliefs like chairs rather tables, because it illustrates how foundationally supportive (or unsupportive) they are to our own selves and experience. The legs of the chair are what give it support to stand, and in the same way your beliefs are supported by evidence and interpretations from your life. The evidence gives your beliefs "legs". When you gather enough evidence to support your limiting belief, you give it legs. The "because" statements you wrote in step 4 are the "legs" of your limiting belief.

6. Break down the legs that support your limiting belief. Think like a lawyer and look for evidence that casts doubt upon or disproves the current evidence supporting your limiting beliefs.

    For example, in my previous statement, "I'm nervous for my talk because… I'm afraid I might not give valuable or inspiring information", I can find evidence to the contrary: "I've spoken about this topic on podcasts and coaching sessions with clients. I'm passionate about it, I enjoy it, and I've received positive feedback about the information I shared."

Your turn:

_____
_____
_____

7. Next, link your limiting belief to some painful or negative consequence in your life. What is that belief costing you in the past, present, or future?

    _____
    _____

"Put blinders on to the things that conspire to hold you back, especially the ones in your own head."

— Meryl Streep

Hooray, you have now dismantled that limiting belief! Now that you've eliminated some of your limiting beliefs and stories, you need new and empowering ones to take their place.

Let's talk about how to create a new belief. Remember how, if beliefs are like a chair, the legs of your beliefs are the references or evidence you use to support it. This supporting evidence is what gives beliefs their structure and allows them to exist at all.

Why do our stories seem so real? It's important to understand that it's not that your beliefs are objectively true, it's just that they *seem* true to you. Let me walk you through an exercise that will demonstrate on a very small scale why your beliefs seem so real to you. Ok, here it goes: Look around you right now, wherever you are, and count how many blue items you see in your field of vision. Any shade of blue works. How many blue items did you count? I bet you saw far more blue things than you had previously noticed before this exercise. It's not that they weren't there before, it's just that you didn't see them because you weren't looking for them.

It's kind of like that with beliefs. When you accept something as true, your brain immediately goes to work to find more evidence that supports it. Psychology offers us an explanation for this phenomenon: it's called confirmation bias. This is basically the tendency to search for, interpret, and recall information in a way that confirms your preexisting beliefs or theories. This illustrates a defining characteristic of beliefs: they are self-reinforcing. Your brain will interpret almost any new information in such a way that it confirms and maintains the belief. Beliefs become self-fulfilling prophecies that perpetuate a cycle of the same results.

Your job is to recognize the beliefs and stories that are out of alignment with who you want to become and integrate new, empowering stories into your life that serve you better.

8. Look back at the list of areas where you feel stuck, and ask yourself, "What would I need to believe in order to succeed here?" Usually, identifying the opposite of your limiting beliefs will help you come up with some empowering ones.

    _____

    _____

    One of the ways you broke down the legs of your limiting beliefs was by finding evidence that contradicted them. Now, give new legs to the empowering beliefs that you've written down. If you've ever made the mistake of Googling symptoms when you felt ill, you probably found that whatever condition you suspected yourself to have, you undoubtedly found information that supported that hypothesis. And the more you searched the internet, the more convinced you became that you had the condition you originally suspected. This is classic confirmation bias – the tendency to search for, interpret, and recall information in a way that confirms your preexisting beliefs, assumptions, and theories. The good news is that you can actually use this principle to your advantage. You can use it to help you come up with evidence to support your empowering beliefs. You can create new beliefs about virtually anything if you find enough evidence to support it.

9. Build the "legs" of your new belief by finding reference or evidence to support it. Simply list all the supporting evidence you can think of.

    _____

    _____

10. Next, link pleasure to your new belief. How will it benefit or improve your circumstances in the present and in the future?

_____

_____

Continue this entire process as many times as needed to firmly and permanently embed it in your brain and psyche. You may want to write it down as a mantra, and rewrite or repeat it many times a day for several days in a row. Repetition is powerful.

Let's look at a few more examples. Let's say you have the limiting belief that your clinic won't be successful because there's too much competition. And let's say you want to adopt the empowering belief that your authenticity is your competitive advantage. How would you do this? You'd start by thinking of times in your life when being authentic has given you an edge or helped you in some way.

Let's look at another new belief. Let's say you have the limiting belief that you need a lot of money to build a business, and this is keeping you from moving forward. Let's say you want to adopt the empowering belief that you don't need a lot of money to build a business because you're resourceful. Here are some references you might use to support this belief: I can use social media to promote my business and get patients. I can start small and keep costs low at first. I can use free services to build a website myself. A woman I know started a successful business with no money. Come to think of it, Apple, Amazon and many other successful companies were started in a garage with little to no capital. See how these references act as supporting legs to your belief chair?

May you have the courage to
break the patterns in your life
that are no longer serving you

The more references you have, the stronger your belief will be. It's just a matter of looking for those references. Remember, you can find evidence to support almost anything if you look hard enough. I recommend writing down all of your supporting references so you can go back and look at them later. The goal is to collect as much evidence as you possibly can that supports your new belief in any way. You're looking for big pieces of evidence, small pieces of evidence, and anything in between. You want to have as many legs on your belief chair as possible. The more legs you have, the stronger the belief will be, and the greater chance it has of sticking.

What helps with my inner critic, in hopes it may help you too

I definitely have some deep-rooted insecurities that continually bubble up - thoughts like, "Who am I to do this?" But I now have the skills to move past these thoughts more easily. And I think that my perseverance in working past my inner critic is a massive contributor to my success.

For example, when sitting down to work on this book, the thought will often arise, "Who am I to write a book to guide my fellow acupuncturist? Who gave me permission? I'm not a millionaire. I don't have multiple locations or a franchise…" When I feel this popping up for me, I know I have to actively select new, more productive thoughts. I'm an acupuncturist who has created the practice of my dreams, what many acupuncturists would also like to create and are struggling to create: a waitlist practice treating two patients an hour so that I can work efficiently while also spending significant time with my patients, associates on staff so that I can take vacations and maternity leave and have freedom in my life, and a steady stream of new patients without spending time or money on marketing so that I can focus on doing what I love. And I have a tested system, philosophy, and approach that

217

I've been able to teach and coach acupuncturists through to predictably produce success for them. I have to continue reminding myself of this truth, and sometimes, I'm my own biggest cheerleader (in response to being my own worst critic – balance :o). The lesson: proactively look for and remind yourself of the evidence that will lift you up and keep you moving towards your dreams.

The inner critic is always loudest right before the breakthrough

I've personally found that my inner critic gets the loudest and meanest whenever I'm asking myself to expand, "uplevel," or do something brave and out of my comfort zone. My best girlfriends now, whenever I share with them that I'm battling my inner critic, automatically ask me what big thing I'm up to or working on. And it's no coincidence - that's exactly when our inner critic typically rears her mean head. Now, I (and my girlfriends) know to expect it. And I can warmly welcome her and accept her presence. The lesson: expect your inner critic to get louder whenever you're about to move towards growth and embrace her.

Something that helps me to determine whether it's my ego/inner critic talking or my intuition/inner sage talking is to quiet myself, get centered in my breathing, tune in, and take notice. Is it a fast, frantic, harsh voice or is it a calm and supportive voice? Our intuition, even when guiding us to say "no" and to maintain boundaries, usually does so in a supportive and calm way: "This isn't for you right now, and that's ok" sort of thing. Whereas our inner critic tends to sound harsh, scared and bossy. Choose to listen to and follow the voice that encourages you to move in the direction of your dreams.

Simply becoming aware of your thoughts is empowering because it allows you to do something about them. Whenever I catch myself thinking negatively, I first become aware of it, and I even name it. My girlfriends and I call my mean inner critic "Nancy", haha, but it can also be helpful to simply call it the Imposter Syndrome or your Inner Critic. Naming it reminds me that it's not really ME or MY TRUTH that's speaking; it's separate from me.

Next, I stop that line of thinking by literally saying, "Stop" to myself really firmly and out loud (people nearby probably think I'm crazy, but oh well). Then, I work on shifting my perspective, questioning my beliefs, and exploring my fears.

One of the biggest fears that holds us back is the fear of being judged. It's helpful for me to remember that we all have this because we're social animals. Our survival for centuries has depended on our ability to fit in with and rely on a group. I think this is why a fear of being judged runs so deep for us. We all have it. We just need to accept and acknowledge it, and continue to move on, speak our truth, and live as authentically as we can. As Brené Brown teaches, our fear of judgement can actually prevent us from achieving what we desire. Ironically, the more vulnerable and true we are, the more able we are to be truly seen, loved, and accepted.

When you feel this fear holding you back, step into being of service – even if it's just to one person. People will be forced to judge you for being of service, helping others, and doing what you love unless you continue to choose to let this fear of being judged hold you back. The real secret to overcoming fear is love. Be love-motivated to serve and share and stay focused on the people you are trying to help. People will sense your genuine intention to be of service and they will be attracted to you. Love does that.

"Life doesn't demand perfection. It doesn't require you to be constantly fearless, confident, or self-assured. It simply requires that you keep showing up."

— Marie Forleo

Chapter 13

Go Forth and Prosper

Being in private practice is a work of heart. It's not just waiting for us. We create it. And while it's daunting and difficult at times, there is a real gift in it.

So many of us came to acupuncture to heal ourselves, and I believe that for many of us, building a practice is an extension of that healing. For me, building a practice has been one of the best "self-help" tools around. It's forced me to confront my inner demons, limiting beliefs, insecurities, and weaknesses. It's forced me to look at places in myself that need attention. The moment I open up to those areas and address them, it shows up in my practice.

It was a struggle for me at first, but I eventually learned to embrace this reality. As a direct result of growing my practice and being forced to confront my weaknesses and put myself and my beliefs out there for the world, I'm now able to more easily recognize what authenticity looks like for me. I'm more and more ok with recognizing my inadequacies as well as my strengths. And I'm able to take that into the treatment room, and into the rest of my life as well. I'm able to feel a sense of alignment, purpose, and confidence that I never knew was possible for me. I feel so grateful for that.

Being in business for yourself and in the service of others invites you to be your most creative, best, authentic, and true self; it requires constant personal reflection and spiritual growth. It's so important to keep working on who we are. We all know that healing takes time. How soon will you step into your power and your confidence? How soon will you own the fact that you're a business owner, a creative, a visionary, and a leader, as well as a healer?

"The best marketing step you could ever take is to be present and inspired with whatever you're doing and whomever you're with. Enthusiastic energy is one of the most radiant and magnetic of all forces. When you love yourself and become inspired, so will others. Marketing is a test of how much inspiration, self-love, and other-love you have, as well as your ability and confidence in communicating it."

— John Demartini

"Knowing is not enough,
we must apply.
willing is not enough,
we must do."

— Bruce Lee

What helped me:

Gratitude

Every day, I make a conscious effort to think of three things I'm most grateful for – whether it's my cozy home, my passion and purpose that light me up, my loving family, or the simple fact that I'm alive. I spend a minute or two first thing in the morning and last thing before I go to bed feeling the gratitude in my body. When I started doing this, I noticed a shift in my life. I felt happier and more empowered, and life flowed more easily.

Throwing pennies for the *I Ching* always helps me to remember to control less and trust more, and to tap into my inner sage.

Don't carry your mistakes around with you. Sometimes, you have to go wrong in order to learn how to go right. And that's ok. It's part of the journey.

Enjoy the journey and celebrate your wins. Whether they're big, small or tiny, enjoy your wins and feel good about them. Share your success with a friend. Do a happy dance. Be proud of yourself.

Take care of yourself. Taking care of yourself is an essential part of taking care of others. The healthier the tree, the better the fruit it can offer. Make time for self-care. Have firm boundaries. I'll be honest, there were times when I struggled with this a lot.

Take action. It's the action you take that will open your eyes and heart, allowing the clarity and confidence to unfold.

"And then I learned the spiritual journey had nothing to do with being nice. It was about being real, authentic. Having boundaries. Honoring my space first, others second. And in this space of self-care being nice just happened, it flowed not motivated by fear but by love"

— Michelle Olak

In review. Don't forget how much demand there is for our services, and how much the world needs us, now more than ever. Embrace the fact that bridging the gap to success requires learning how to communicate the value of your services so that people see the specific value in it for them. Aim to serve and contribute and champion others' wins as much as your own. Be yourself. Be authentic. Don't sell out. Sow your seeds consistently, build your authority, focus on the long game and nurture relationships. Think of yourself as an authority, dose your medicine appropriately, and learn to step into your confidence and power. These are my wishes for you. A rising tide lifts all that float, and we, my friend, are rising.

I want to remind you again how amazing acupuncture is. People love getting acupuncture because they walk out feeling better. How often can you say that about a regular doctor appointment? And when done with the appropriate frequency, it can have transformative and lasting effects. AND their symptoms aren't just improved - they also feel heard, cared for, empowered, and prepared, and they understand themselves a little better. Our medicine, and you, are amazing, my friend. I feel so honored. So amazed. So grateful to my patients and to this medicine. So lucky to get walk with people on their healing journeys.

We are all special. We are all worthy. We are all capable of greatness. We are all equal. Because we are all here. And I believe we are here for a reason. I believe you're here for a reason. Tune in to your intuition. Trust yourself. The world needs you. The world is ready for you, now more than ever.

We've come to the end of our journey together in this book. I'd like to honor and thank you for being here, reading this, and being you. Getting this book out of my head and onto paper has been challenging, and I resisted it, but it feels well worth it to have sidelined my resistance and gone for it. My hope is that it will help to inspire you to go for your dreams too.

If you enjoyed this book, please reach out to me and let me know. I would love hearing from you. Leave a review to let other acupuncturists know if you found it helpful, and pass it along to a friend so that we can continue to lift each other up. Because we are rising, my friend, together!

If you'd like more education and support, check out all the resources available on acuprosper.com. I offer free and paid courses, group coaching programs, and one-on-one hourly coaching "jam sessions" designed to lift you up, show you the ropes, and provide you with a supportive community of like-minded acupuncturists.

Every person reading this is a light-worker with a mission. You are here to rise up and honor why you're here so that you can be of service to every being that you touch; so that you can have an imprint on this world that so desperately needs you. You're wonderful and amazing and I wish you so much success along your beautiful journey.

With so much love,

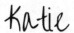

P.S. I made a free gift for you – a guided visualization to support you in growing your practice and confidently and compassionately showing the world (and yourself) that you mean business.

Go to www.acuprosper.com/free-gift to get it.

The ego is never ready.
The soul is always ready.
It's the soul who does the work.

Made in the USA
Monee, IL
10 August 2024

63585767R10134